W0080632

A Guide to
Laboratory Safety and
Microscale Organic
Laboratory Techniques

A Guide to Laboratory Safety and Microscale Organic Laboratory Techniques

Mayura A Kale BPharm, MPharm, PhD
Assistant Professor (Pharm Chemistry)
Government College of Pharmacy
Aurangabad, Maharashtra, India

Satish Y Gabhe BPharm, MPharm, PhD
Professor (Pharm Chemistry)
Bharati Vidyapeeth's Poona College of Pharmacy
Pune, Maharashtra, India

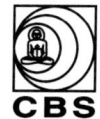

CBS

CBS Publishers & Distributors Pvt Ltd

New Delhi • Bengaluru • Chennai • Kochi • Kolkata • Mumbai

Bhopal • Bhubaneswar • Hyderabad • Jharkhand • Nagpur • Patna • Pune • Uttarakhand • Dhaka (Bangladesh)

Disclaimer

Science and technology are constantly changing fields. New research and experience broaden the scope of information and knowledge. The authors have tried their best in giving information available to them while preparing the material for this book. Although all efforts have been made to ensure optimum accuracy of the material, yet it is quite possible some errors might have been left uncorrected. The publisher, the printer and the authors will not be held responsible for any inadvertent errors or inaccuracies.

A Guide to
Laboratory Safety and
Microscale Organic
Laboratory Techniques

ISBN: 978-93-88178-92-1

Copyright © Authors and Publisher

First Edition: 2019

All rights reserved. No part of this book may be reproduced or transmitted in any form or by any means, electronic or mechanical, including photocopying, recording, or any information storage and retrieval system without permission, in writing, from the authors and the publisher.

Published by Satish Kumar Jain and Produced by Varun Jain for

CBS Publishers & Distributors Pvt Ltd
4819/XI Prahlad Street, 24 Ansari Road, Daryaganj, New Delhi 110 002, India.
Ph: 23289259, 23266861, 23266867   Fax: 011-23243014   Website: www.cbspd.com
                                                              e-mail: delhi@cbspd.com; cbspubs@airtelmail.in.
Corporate Office: 204 FIE, Industrial Area, Patparganj, Delhi 110 092
Ph: 4934 4934   Fax: 4934 4935   e-mail: publishing@cbspd.com; publicity@cbspd.com

Branches

- **Bengaluru:** Seema House 2975, 17th Cross, K.R. Road,
  Banasankari 2nd Stage, Bengaluru 560 070, Karnataka
  Ph: +91-80-26771678/79   Fax: +91-80-26771680   e-mail: bangalore@cbspd.com
- **Chennai:** 7, Subbaraya Street, Shenoy Nagar, Chennai 600 030, Tamil Nadu
  Ph: +91-44-26680620, 26681266   Fax: +91-44-42032115   e-mail: chennai@cbspd.com
- **Kochi:** 42/1325, 1326, Power House Road, Opp. KSEB Power House
  Ernakulam 682 018, Kochi, Kerala
  Ph: +91-484-4059061-65   Fax: +91-484-4059065   e-mail: kochi@cbspd.com
- **Kolkata:** 6/B, Ground Floor, Rameswar Shaw Road, Kolkata-700 014, West Bengal
  Ph: +91-33-22891126, 22891127, 22891128   e-mail: kolkata@cbspd.com
- **Mumbai:** 83-C, Dr E Moses Road, Worli, Mumbai-400018, Maharashtra
  Ph: +91-22-24902340/41   Fax: +91-22-24902342   e-mail: mumbai@cbspd.com

Representatives

• Bhopal	0-8319310552	• Bhubaneswar	0-9911037372	• Hyderabad	0-9885175004
• Jharkhand	0-9811541605	• Nagpur	0-9421945513	• Patna	0-9334159340
• Pune	0-9623451994	• Uttarakhand	0-9716462459	• Dhaka (Bangladesh)	01912-003485

Printed at Glorious Printers, Daryaganj, Delhi, India

Preface

Microscale chemistry has been often referred to as small-scale chemistry. Pioneering development in this area was carried out by Egerton C Grey, Mahmoud K El-Marsafy in Egypt and Stephen Thompson in the USA. Further application of these ideas was devised by Bradley (of the Radmaste kits) in South Africa. It was designed to make effective chemical experiments possible in developing countries in schools having shortage of chemicals and funds. Another way is introducing this approach into synthetic work, mainly in organic chemistry. Here, the crucial breakthrough was achieved by Mayo, Pike, Butcher and Williamson who demonstrated that inexperienced students could carry out organic synthesis on a few tenths of milligrams, a skill previously thought to require years of training and experience. These approaches were accompanied by the introduction of some specialized equipment subsequently simplified by Breuer without great loss of versatility.

This approach is now adopted worldwide. It has become a major presence on the educational scene in the United States, used to a lesser extent in the United Kingdom, and used in many countries in institutions with faculties who are enthusiastic about it.

Mayura A Kale
Satish Y Gabhe

Acknowledgements

I express my sincere gratitude to respected Dr VK Mourya, Principal, Government College of Pharmacy, Aurangabad, Maharashtra, who has been a source of inspiration and who ignited the spark of concept of microscale chemistry in me.

I would also appreciate the support of my PhD student Mr Gajanan Sonwane and MPharm–Pharm Chem (2015–2017) batch students for supporting me in performing microscale techniques and experiments before I could pen these down in the form of this book.

I also express my thanks to the concerned staff members of CBS Publishers & Distributors Pvt Ltd for putting exhaustive efforts in publishing this book.

Mayura A Kale

Contents

Introduction

Microscale chemistry has been often referred to as small-scale chemistry. It is not only an analytical and synthetic method, but also a teaching method widely used at school and university level, working with small quantities of chemical substances. Pioneering development in this area was carried out by Egerton C Grey, Mahmoud K El-Marsafy in Egypt, Stephen Thompson in the US and others. A further application of these ideas was devised by Bradley of the Radmaste kits in South Africa. It was designed to make effective chemical experiments possible in developing countries in schools having shortage of chemicals and funds. Another way is the introduction of this approach into synthetic work, mainly in organic chemistry. Here, the crucial breakthrough was achieved by Mayo, Pike and Butcher and by Williamson who demonstrated that inexperienced students were able to carry out organic syntheses on a few tenths of milligrams, a skill previously thought to require years of training and experience. These approaches were accompanied by the introduction of some specialized equipment, subsequently simplified by Breuer without great loss of versatility. This approach is now adopted worldwide. It has become a major presence on the educational scene in the United States, used to a lesser extent in the United Kingdom, and used in many countries in institutions with faculties who are enthusiastic about it.

With the attributes and benefits of microscale organic synthesis discussed previously, it is not surprising that it has spread like wildfire mainly in developing countries, including India. It has also developed profound roots throughout the world which will make the tree grow quite high for the years to come. Both developed and underdeveloped countries will continue benefiting from this approach. There are many other advantages of combining microscale chemistry with green chemistry and microwave-assisted organic synthesis because all of these have a common objective of reducing chemical risks. Together, all these techniques represent an effective approach to education and training in chemistry at all levels. Also, advances in current experimental organic chemistry can be achieved and skills can be developed by hands on experience by using special equipment, methods and studying reactions at a more deeper level. This technique shall also become a landmark for scale-up of intermediates and reagents in the research and development. The beneficiaries of this book include undergraduate as well as postgraduate students of pharmacy as well as BSc and MSc (organic chemistry).

The progress in current experimental organic chemistry shall become easy after gaining expertise in microscale techniques. In this book, introduction to the special equipment used in microscale experiments, as well as different methods which are used, will be presented. It will also enable the students in developing skills needed to study organic reactions at a deeper and detailed level. Microscale chemistry has developed and created revolution in chemical educational reforms. It has opened various avenues for quality education and has motivated the imaginative power, responsiveness and skills of students towards environmental protection. It has also deterred the reputation of organic chemistry laboratory of being malodorous and hazardous. Since, the advent of microscale techniques in industries and academia, many reactions could be carried out safely with many additional benefits. It has made organic chemistry more fulfilling and a rewarding experience.

The book journey starts with exemplifying the importance of laboratory safety in laboratory. This is a very important aspect that the students must be made aware of before the start of any experiment. The related matter has been written in a simple and lucid way. Usually one is familiar with the traditional methodologies of working in an organic chemistry laboratory at macro- and semi-microscale level. The microscale organic chemistry techniques shall enhance the existing skills of an individual for better understanding. Extremely small amounts of chemicals will be handled. Most of the researchers and students will find it interesting.

Traditionally, experiments in organic chemistry are carried out on a macroscale level, employing quantities of chemicals on the order of 5–100 g, using glassware designed to contain between 25 and 500 ml of liquids. For quantities of materials in the 0.005–0.5 gram range, one employs different technique called "microscale" in order to carry out various standard organic laboratory operations. The students at this point are introduced with the microscale apparatus and techniques. In the next chapter, the practical applications of microscale techniques in the form of medicinal organic synthesis are given. Last, the importance of combinations of microscale with microwave technique and green chemistry is highlighted. We wish that this book becomes a landmark for undergraduate and postgraduate students studying pharmacy and organic chemistry .

CHAPTER 1

Organic Chemistry Laboratory and Safety Procedures

1. ORGANIC CHEMISTRY LABORATORY—WORKING

The progress in current experimental organic chemistry shall become easier after gaining expertise in microscale techniques. In this book, introduction to the special equipment used in microscale experiments, as well as different methods which are used, are presented. It will also enable the students in developing skills needed to study organic reactions at a more deeper and detailed level. Microscale chemistry has developed and created revolution in chemical educational reforms. It has opened various avenues for quality education and has motivated the imaginative power, responsiveness and skills of students towards environmental protection. It has also deterred the reputation of organic chemistry laboratory of being malodorous and hazardous. Since, the advent of microscale techniques in industries and academia, many reactions could be carried out safely with many additional benefits. It has made organic chemistry more fulfilling and a rewarding experience. Usually one is familiar with the traditional methodologies of working in an organic chemistry laboratory at macro- and semi-micro level. The microscale organic chemistry techniques shall enhance the existing skills of an individual for better understanding. In these techniques, extremely small amounts of chemicals will be handled and most of the researchers and students will find it interesting.

1

Following are some of the important points to be followed while working in an organic chemistry laboratory:

a. **Understanding the experiment before performing it in laboratory:** This is one of the most important prerequisite before carrying out actual experiment. One must know exactly what is to be done. Occasionally incomplete directions or a misunderstanding of instructions causes accidents. Whenever in doubt, do not hesitate to ask for the correct way of doing the experiment. While performing microscale organic experiments, various unit operations take place very speedily in comparison to macroscale experiments. Hence, getting familiar with the various processes in advance will prove to be beneficial. In addition to this, various techniques adopted in microscale experiments are critical and need hands on experience to attain expertise. If proper study of the experimental sequences has not been done before starting it, then it can create chaos and break attentiveness. It might also lead to some untoward incidence.

b. **Weighing and measuring of quantities:** In microscale experiments, the quantities used are less than a gram of starting materials and volumes less than a few mililitres. It is therefore very important to weigh and measure the quantities used in such microscale experiments more carefully and accurately. This will considerably reduce the quantitation-related errors.

c. **Use of clean equipment:** The importance of proper cleaning of equipment must be appreciated because contaminated equipment is a major cause of reaction failure, lower yields and impure products. It increases time required for further purification of product and results in cost escalation. One must devote time to clean the equipment properly, before starting the experiment.

d. **Storage of the reaction flasks when not in use:** The reaction flasks used in microscale technique are small in size and should be placed in an appropriate sized container, usually a beaker when not in use. This is done so as to avoid accidental spillage of its contents. This can cause damage to the work place, injury to individuals, waste of time and money (if the reactants are expensive). If the flask is kept in a beaker, these problems can be avoided and the product can be recovered.

e. **Use of clean and dry glassware:** It is necessary to clean and dry glassware as soon as possible prior to storage. Dirty glassware is harder to clean after some time and spoils further experimentation. It may become unusable and will have to be discarded.

f. **Experimentation on a clean laboratory bench surface:** Work surfaces such as laboratory benches must be cleaned before and after experimentation.

g. **Discarding of chemicals:** Do not discard anything unless one is sure that it is not harmful and will not be required in future experiments. Generally, different solvents should be discarded separately in different solvent containers.

h. **Supporting round-bottom flasks containing liquid reaction mixtures:** In some reactions containing liquids, internal pressure may increase and can cause bumping of the reaction mixture; sometimes along with loss of material. Such reactions should be carefully stirred or porcelain chips should be used while heating.

Any reaction with volatile liquids should not be carried out in an air tight container. This has large potential for explosive accidents (unless it is stored in a well-sealed pressure vessel) due to increase in the pressure.

2. GENERAL PRECAUTIONS

Organic chemistry can be a gratifying and pleasant experience, but it can also be dangerous. Improper judgement in the laboratory is one of the major reasons for several accidents that occur in it. Hence, it is mandatory to stick to the procedures outlined in the experiment and follow the good laboratory practices. The scientific spirit of experimentation and exploration has made many wonderful discoveries, but it has also got a lot of people hurt or killed in the past in order to discover what is safe and what is not! Do not go mixing things just to see what will happen!

I. GENERAL SAFETY/HAZARD WARNING SIGNS (Fig. 1.1)

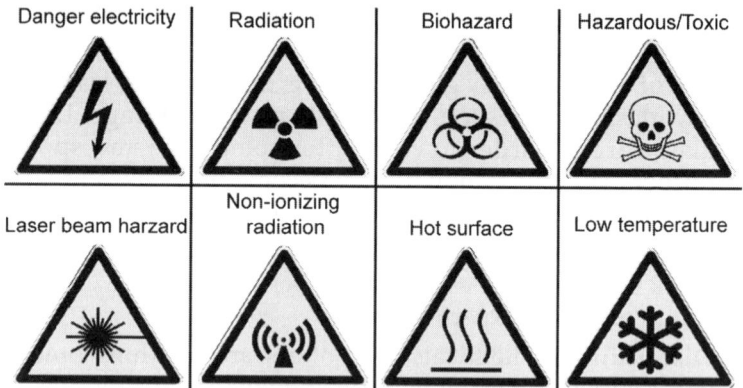

Fig. 1.1: Hazard warning sign

II. CHEMICAL SAFETY SYMBOLS

a. The word "Poison" is often used interchangeably with the word "Toxic" (Fig. 1.2). Most chemicals are fairly dangerous if ingested or inhaled but many of these are dangerous even on contact. Many of these are in aqueous solution, but they are also available as mixtures or pure compounds. For example, acrylamide, formaldehyde, glutaraldehyde, chloroform, phenol, methylene chloride, metal salts such as silver chloride, cadmium sulfate, mercuric acetate, barium carbonate, lead acetate, biological stains, sodium cyanide, potassium cyanide, calcium cyanide, etc.

Fig. 1.2: Poisonous/toxic

b. Environmental hazard is relatively rare with laboratory chemicals and most of them pose environmental hazard if these are not disposed correctly (Fig. 1.3). For example, arsenic salts, mercury salts, etc.

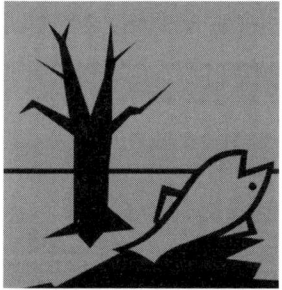

Fig. 1.3: Environmental Hazard

c. Corrosive chemicals cause visible destruction or irreversible alterations in living tissue by chemical action at the site of contact (Fig. 1.4). Hence, it is advised to avoid their contact with skin. These are also known to rust the chemical cupboards under certain conditions. For example, strong acids, strong bases, gases, viz. ammonia, hydrogen chloride, nitrogen dioxide, sulfur dioxide, bromine, amines, hydrofluoric acid, perchloric acid, etc.

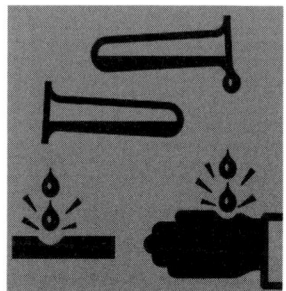

Fig. 1.4: Corrosive

d. Chemicals that are explosives cause a sudden, almost instantaneous release of pressure, gas, and heat when subjected to sudden shock, pressure or high temperature

(Fig. 1.5). These are chemicals that can result in damage to surrounding materials (hoods, glassware, windows, people, etc.) and generating toxic gases and fires. For example, acetyl peroxide, acetylene, ammonium nitrate, ammonium perchlorate, picric acid, picryl chloride, trinitrobenzoic acid, trinitroresorcinol, trinitrotoluene, nitroglycerine, nitroguanidine, trinitroaniline, trinitroanisole, etc.

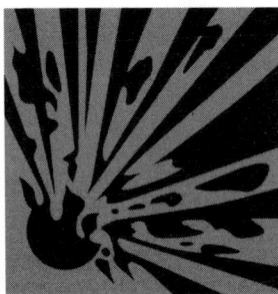

Fig. 1.5: Explosive

e. Flammable chemicals are liquids which give off enough vapors to ignite in the presence of an ignition source at a temperature less than 37.8°C. Such chemicals are to be stored in flame-resistant cupboards. Volatile solvents can be a particular problem as they are prone to spread around from unsealed containers. This also covers pyrophoric materials which catch fire spontaneously on exposure to air. When using flammable liquids, the containers are to be kept away from open flames. It is best to use heating sources such as steam bath, water bath, oil bath, and heating mantel. Never use a heat gun to heat a flammable liquid (Fig. 1.6). For example, methanol, ethanol, acetone, xylenes, toluene, ethyl acetate, tetrahydrofuran, ethyl ether, benzene, dimethylformamide, acetonitrile, hexane, pyridine, glacial acetic acid (100%), acetic acid (>80%), acetic anhydride, formic acid (>85%), propanoic acid (100%), triethylamine, diethylamine, ethylaminediamine, trimethylamine solution, pyrrolidine, morpholine, cyclohexylamine, etc.

Fig. 1.6: Flammable or extremely flammable

f. Irritant substances are those chemicals which cause inflammation and pain at the site of contact with skin and other tissues (Fig. 1.7). This symbol covers a wide range of relatively minor hazards. However, precautions such as avoid contact with the skin, do not breathe, etc. should be scrupulously followed. For example, acetonitrile, chloroform, dimethyl sulphoxide, formaldehyde, sodium azide, sodium hydroxide, sodium hypochlorite, tetrahydrofuran, etc.

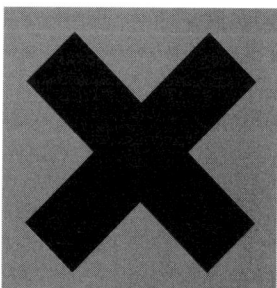

Fig. 1.7: Irritant or harmful

g. Oxidising chemicals are those that are other than blasting agents or explosives that initiate or promote combustion in other materials, thereby causing fire either of itself or through the release of oxygen or other gases (Fig. 1.8). These are known to spontaneously evolve oxygen at room temperature or with slight heating, or that promote combustion. These are to be kept away from flammable chemicals at all costs. For example, inorganic nitrates, nitrites, permanganates, chlorates, perchlorates, iodates, periodates, persulfates, chromates, hypochlorites, peroxides, potassium perchlorate, calcium hypochlorite, sodium nitrate, sodium iodate, ammonium persulfate, sodium peroxide, etc.

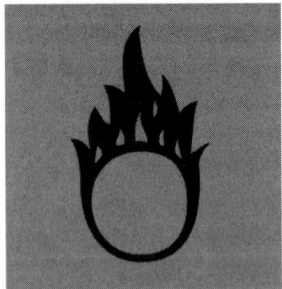

Fig. 1.8: Oxidizing chemical

h. Dangerous chemicals are those which react violently with water to form toxic vapors and/or flammable gases that can ignite and cause fire. This symbol generally means that it will react fairly violently with water. Any paper toweling, gloves, etc. that have come into contact with these materials need to be quenched with water before disposing of in metal trash cans in order to prevent potential fires (Fig. 1.9). For example, sodium metal, salts of sodium, calcium, potassium, calcium with carbides, etc.

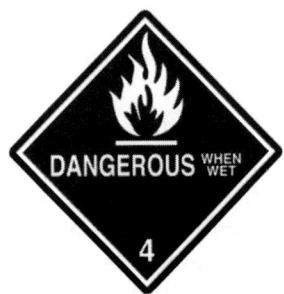

Fig. 1.9: Dangerous when wet

i. Organic peroxides are compounds that contain bivalent – O-O- structure and which may be considered to be structural derivatives of hydrogen peroxide where one or both of the hydrogen atoms have been replaced by an organic radical (Fig. 1.10). Oxidizers and organic peroxides are a concern for laboratory safety due to their ability to promote and enhance the potential for fires in laboratories. This chemical safety symbol indicates the transport and storage of organic peroxides. For example, hydrogen peroxide, peroxy acids, etc.

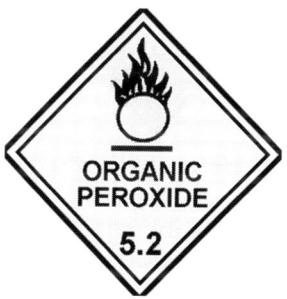

Fig. 1.10: Organic peroxide

j. Flammable solids are solids other than blasting agents or explosives which are liable to cause fire through friction, absorption of moisture, spontaneous chemical change, or retained heat from manufacturing or processing, or which can be ignited readily and when ignited, burn so vigorously and persistently to create a serious hazard (Fig. 1.11). For example, sodium metal, benzoquinone, 2,4-dinitrophenyl hydrazine, 2,4-dinitrophenol, benzoyl peroxide, maleic acid, etc.

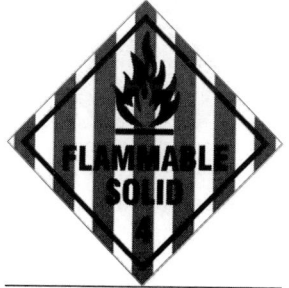

Fig. 1.11: Flammable solid

k. This is the safety symbol used in the transport of non-flammable gases and hence often non-hazardous, at least out in the open (Fig. 1.12). For example, ammonia, argon, carbon dioxide, hydrogen halides, krypton, sulphur dioxide, etc.

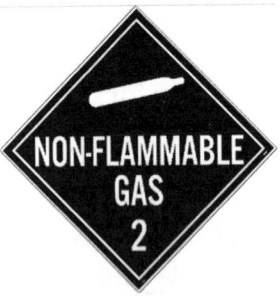

Fig. 1.12: Non-flammable gas

l. Spontaneously combustible materials are also known as pyrophorics (Fig. 1.13). These chemicals can spontaneously ignite in the presence of air, some are reactive with water vapor, and most are reactive with oxygen. Extra care must be taken when handling spontaneously combustible chemicals. When transporting these chemicals, it is best to use a bottle carrier and carts. For example, tertiary butyl lithium, white phosphorus, etc.

Fig. 1.13: Spontaneously combustible

m. This symbol is used for the transport or storage of chemicals which are hazardous to inhale (Fig. 1.14).

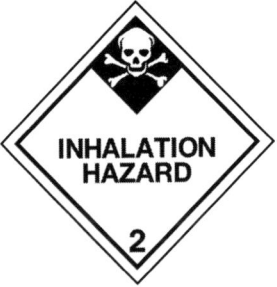

Fig. 1.14: Inhalation hazard

n. This symbol is used for the transport of a poisonous gas - on gas cylinders, or sometimes as an indicator on vehicles (Fig. 1.15).

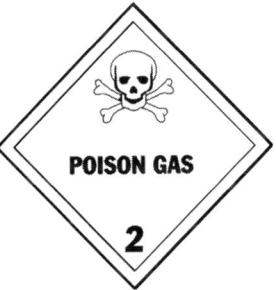

Fig. 1.15: Poisonous gas

o. This symbol indicates that harmful material should be kept away from edible material (Fig. 1.16).

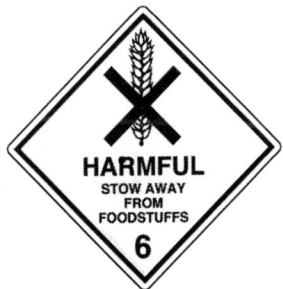

Fig. 1.16: Stow away from foodstuffs

p. This is the safety symbol used for the transport or storage of a flammable gas (Fig. 1.17).

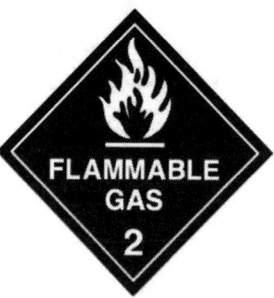

Fig. 1.17: Flammable gas

q. This is a catch-all symbol for all other dangers (Fig. 1.18).

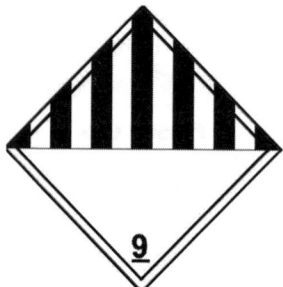

Fig. 1.18: Miscellaneous danger

III. SAFETY RULES TO BE FOLLOWED IN LABORATORY

1. **Procedure for reporting the accidents in laboratory:** One should report such cases to the lab-incharge or head of department. The reporting should be done even if the injury appears to be minor. Always cooperate with the people around oneself.

2. **Precautions and care during experimentation:** There are fair chances of eyes getting severely damaged due to flying broken glass pieces or due to spillage of chemicals. It is a good practice to wear safety goggles all the time in the laboratory.

3. **Use of safety gloves:** These are to be used when working with highly toxic, corrosive, caustic or allergenic, carcinogenic, mutagenic and teratogenic compounds. These also provide protection against some toxic solvents which may deeply penetrate the skin and cause damage. Unfortunately, wearing safety gloves does not give universal protection, but do provide substantial protection against a wide range of chemicals.

4. **Proper use of glassware:** The most common injuries that occur in chemistry laboratories are cuts and burns.

   Such injuries can be prevented by following a few simple rules:

   a. When inserting glass tubing into rubber stoppers, make sure the glass tubing ends are fire polished (very smooth and rounded).

   b. Always use lubricant such as glycerin or soapy water on the inside of any tubing and on the outside of glass. Protect the hand by wrapping the glass tubing with a towel.

   c. Hold the glass near the end to be inserted, thus minimizing the torque, and insert using twisting motion and never hold the glass at a bend.

   d. Be careful with glassware that is "frozen." Only after wearing goggles and gloves, one should try to release such "frozen" glassware and if this fails, discard the glassware. Some common cases of "frozen" glassware include nested beakers that have been jammed together, stoppers that cannot be removed from bottles and also the stopcocks that cannot be moved.

   e. Discard cracked or broken glassware in the designated container which should be clearly labeled "broken glassware only". When handling broken glassware, wear gloves or use a dustpan and broom and do not pick up broken glass with bare hands.

   f. Never heat heavy glassware such as graduated cylinders, suction flasks, or reagent bottles since they might shatter.

   g. Never set hot glassware on cold surfaces or in any way change its temperature suddenly.

5. **Procedure in case of chemical spills**

   a. If one receives a chemical burn from a caustic material, i.e. acid or base, immediately wash the area with large quantities of water continuously for a few minutes under a running tap. Ask another student to inform the lab-in-charge.

   b. Wash the hands and face quickly and thoroughly whenever they come into contact with a chemical.

   c. Always wash the hands, before leaving the lab since toxic chemicals may be ingested at a later time via hands.

   d. Chemicals spilled over a large part of the body require immediate attention. Remove all the contaminated clothing and use the safety shower, flooding the affected area. Do not use creams and lotions, but instead get immediate medical attention.

6. **Care with flames:** One of the major fire hazard can be a lighted gas burner.

   a. Safety measures to be followed are:
      - The burner should be burning only for the period of time in which it is actually used.
      - Before lighting the burner carefully position it on the desk away from flammable materials, reagent shelves, flammable or low boiling chemicals/solvents/reagents (acetone, toluene, alcohol, etc.).
      - Be careful not to extend your arm over a burner while reaching for something.

   b. Personal precautions to be followed are:
      - Keep long hair tied back or put inside lab coat so that it will not catch fire.
      - Keep long beards away from flames.

7. **Do not point a test tube toward a laboratory neighbor or yourself:** This is to be followed when heating a reaction mixture in a test tube over a burner.

8. **Wear appropriate clothing:** Wear clothing that will protect oneself against spilled chemicals or flaming liquids. A standard lab coat is usually sufficient. Hard-soled, covered footwear must be worn in the laboratory at all times and sandals should not be worn.

9. **Presumption of a particular reagent being hazardous**
   a. Never taste a chemical unless specifically directed to do so.
   b. If one is instructed to smell a chemical, point the vessel away from the face and carefully fan the vapors toward your face with your hand and sniff gently.
   c. Material Safety Data Sheets (MSDS) should be available for every chemical used in the laboratory. This document is used internationally and has information about the chemical, physical, and physiological properties of chemical substances, various health hazards, how to clean up spills, fire danger, and what to do if one is exposed to the chemical. A shortcut to MSDS websites should be made available through laboratory computers. They can also be found by entering the name of the chemical and MSDS into authentic internet search engine.

10. **Avoid mouth-pipetting:** Avoid this to keep internal organs such as trachea, lungs, GIT, free from injury or abnormal exposure to toxic vapours/liquids.

11. **Assemble safe apparatus:** Always put together an apparatus as outlined in the instructions. Grease the ground glass joints with silicone grease. Poor apparatus assemblies are the first steps to an accident.

12. **Dilute concentrated acids/alkalies:** Do not pour water into concentrated acids/alkalies, as most of the time, it is an exothermic reaction. The heat evolved will cause the water to boil and spill all over the place along with the acid.

13. **Use of fume hoods:** Fume hoods protect the user from inhaling toxic or poisonous gases and also protect the product or experiment. These also keep the environment safe when fitted with appropriate filters in the exhaust airstream. Fume hoods function by drawing the air inside from the front open side of the cabinet in the laboratory and either expelling it outside the building or made safe through filtration and fedback into the laboratory.

14. **Read the labels:** Read the labels carefully before taking anything from a bottle. Many chemicals have similar names, such as sodium nitrate and sodium nitrite. Using

the wrong reagent can spoil an experiment or can cause a serious accident.

15. **Strictly prohibited activities in the laboratory must be avoided:** Eating, drinking and smoking are the activities to be strictly prohibited in the laboratory. This must be followed at all times because there is a high possibility of chemicals getting into the mouth or lungs through contamination. The chief hazard with smoking is fire.

16. **Place for hot objects:** Do not forget to place hot objects on a wire gauze or ceramic pad. These should not be kept directly on the bench top.

17. **Disposal of lighted matches:** Do not throw the lighted matches into the sink. They may ignite a discarded flammable liquid or some solid chemical already present in the sink and cause fire.

18. **Performing experiments:** Variations in the experiments can be attempted only when permitted do to so. Performing unauthorized experiments is dangerous. Persons lacking the experience to recognize whether or not the chemicals and techniques are safe should never attempt such things.

19. **Maintenance of workspace**
    a. Place tall items, such as graduated cylinders, toward the back of the workbench so they will not be overturned by reaching over them.
    b. Clean up all chemical spills, scraps of paper, and glassware immediately with proper care.
    c. Keep drawers closed while working and the aisles free of any obstructions, including chairs, stools, etc.
    d. Never place coats, books, and other belongings on the laboratory bench where they will interfere with the experiment and are likely to be damaged.
    e. Wash and wipe off the desktop.
    f. Be sure gas and water taps are turned off.
    g. Return all special equipment to the stockroom.
    h. Put everything back into the locker drawer and lock.

20. **Proper use of reagents**
    a. Never use more than the required amount of reagents in the experiment.

b. Do not return any excess chemical to the reagent bottle; share it with another student or dispose it according the instructions listed under 22.

c. If one is uncertain how to dispose of an excess of a specific chemical, consult the lab-incharge before taking chances which may prove dangerous and harmful.

21. Disposal of chemicals

Material/Chemical	Nature of disposal container
Non-flammable, water-soluble liquids	Liquid waste bottle
Chemical solids, contaminated paper and broken glassware	Solid waste bottle
Paper products	Trash can
Organic solvents	Organic waste bottle (do not put acids in the organic waste bottle)
Glass tubing waste or broken glass	Wooden box

22. Proper addition of a reagent: The reasons for this are:

a. Some reactions give off a lot of heat, and unless added slowly, can become too vigorous and go out of control. Do not dump the reagent in the reaction vessel.

b. If one makes a mistake and chooses the wrong chemical, adding slowly decreases the possibility of causing a serious accident.

23. Handling chemical spills

a. Alert everyone in the lab.

b. Clean up the spill as directed by the lab-incharge.

c. Immediate medical attention should be given to the affected person.

24. Attitude in the laboratory: Negligence towards the work in the laboratory should not be allowed as it will finally affect others, spoil the aura and will greatly affect the experimental result.

25. Do not be a sufferer of the lab neighbors' mistakes: Bring to the notice of the lab-incharge if anyone is following unacceptable and unprofessional behavior or improper techniques in the laboratory. This is to be done to prevent mishaps.

26. **Observation of specific precautions and modifications in experiments:** Failure to observe the precautions might lead to disastrous results. Also, timely modifications suggested should be understood and followed to get reproducible experimental results.

27. **Maintenance of inventory of chemicals in the laboratory:** Always maintain an inventory data of chemicals in the respective laboratories and do not misplace or exchange chemicals from one laboratory to another. This is done to avoid chaos when any chemical is required urgently during a specific reaction step.

28. **Punctuality in the laboratory:** One should arrive on time for all laboratory sessions to be present to hear the safety information provided by the lab-incharge. For the safety of all the others in the laboratory, the persons who arrive late should be allowed to perform the experiment that day only after giving proper instructions.

29. **Posters and signs:** Posters highlighting the safety rules and techniques are effective reminders to all who enter the laboratory.

30. **Laboratory hygiene:** One should never eat, drink or smoke in the laboratory. Also, one should never apply cosmetics, touch the face, mouth or eyes, suck pens or chew pencils after entering in the laboratory. One must always wash hands before leaving the laboratory and especially before eating.

31. **Laboratory clothing and footwear:** One should use clothes, which are not too loose, especially at the sleeves. Laboratory coats or aprons must be worn over clothes. Snaps or fasteners are preferable to buttons for quicker removal of clothes in case of an emergency. Also, one must wear shoes that fully cover the feet. Shoes provide a great deal of initial protection in the case of dropped containers, spilled chemicals and unseen hazards on the floor. Tie back long hair so that it will not fall on the flames or chemicals. Exposed body skin gives added risk to irritation and burns by corrosive chemicals and gases.

Aprons usually refer to being made of plastic or rubber, which protect against corrosive and irritating chemicals. Labcoats made of cotton are good for protection against flying objects, sharp or rough edges and usually treated with a fire retardant. If made up of wool, these protect against molten splashes, small acid spills and small flames and if these are of synthetic fibre source, protect against IR and UV radiation but burn easily and can be ruined by strong solvents.

32. **Laboratory first aid kits:** It is recommended that basic first aid kit should contain the following items; one absorbent compress, few adhesive bandages, adhesive tape, individual use antiseptic applications, individual use burn treatment applications, pairs of medical examination gloves, sterile pads, triangular bandage, bandage compresses of various pad sizes, eye covering(s) with the ability to cover both eyes, eyewash (sterile, isotonic, buffered solution in individual use applications), cold pack, gauze roller bandage, adhesive bandages of assorted sizes, plastic bags, scissors with rounded tips, forceps (tweezers), a small flashlight with extra batteries, a blanket, eyewash cups or eye irrigator loops, suction type contact lens remover.

33. **Signs and labels:** Various types of signs and labels should be posted in prominent areas of the laboratory and adjoining area. These include emergency telephone numbers, laboratory safety rules, labels indicating types of hazardous contents of cabinets and in chemical storerooms, the National Fire Protection Association (NFPA) diamond with the highest hazard ratings of the materials in the rooms. In addition, there should be posting of location signs for fire extinguishers, fire blankets, spill kit, goggle cabinet, exits, waste containers (e.g. chemical, broken glass) and gas and electric cut-off points.

IV. PRELIMINARY TRAINING ON USAGE OF SAFETY EQUIPMENT

One should get familiar with the location, uses and method of operation of safety equipment.

1. **Eyewash:** Emergency eyewashes are used when the eyes or face may come into contact with any substance which can

cause corrosion, severe irritation or permanent tissue damage or which is toxic by absorption. Most eyewash have a paddle that activates flow when one leans on it pushing it forward and downward. Help the affected person in holding open the eyelids during flushing. With chemicals in the eye, the eyelids have a natural tendency to close tightly. The eyelids need to be pried open and held open to allow the water to remove the damaging substance.

2. **Face shields:** Full face shields protect the face and neck better than goggles. These shields are not a substitute for chemical splash safety goggles. When maximum protection from flying particles and harmful liquids is needed, face shields should be worn with goggles.

3. **Safety shower:** It is an emergency system used to protect laboratory chemist from injury in case of contact with hazardous chemicals and fire. It should also be used if one suffers a massive spill of a dangerous chemical on oneself and need to get it off rapidly. Proper use of this equipment reduces chances of permanent or severe injury.

   The emergency eyewash and the emergency shower may be used simultaneously. Seek medical advice and attention while the exposed worker remains under the shower and also ask as to how long the exposed laboratory worker should remain under the shower before leaving to seek medical attention and discuss various options for transportation (e.g. ambulance). If unable to obtain this information in a timely manner then the standard rule of thumb is to remain under the shower for 15 minutes.

4. **Fire extinguishers:** These are active fire protection devices used to extinguish or control small fires, often in emergency situations. It is not intended for use on an out-of-control fire, such as one which has reached the ceiling, endangers the user or otherwise requires the expertise of a fire department. Typically, a fire extinguisher consists of a hand-held cylindrical pressure vessel containing an agent which can be discharged to extinguish a fire. These smother the burning material so that it cannot get enough air (oxygen) for the fire to continue to burn, e.g. carbon dioxide, dry chemical and foam fire extinguishers. Also, water-type extinguishers cool

the burning material so much that there is not enough heat to support the fire.

Fires are classified according to the type of fuel that is burning. If one uses the wrong type of fire extinguisher on the wrong class of fire, it can make matters worse. There are four types of fire:

Class A: Wood, paper, cloth, trash, plastic, solid combustible materials that are not metals. (Class A fires generally leave an ash.)

Class B: Flammable liquids: gasoline, oil, grease, acetone, any non-metal in a liquid state, on fire, flammable gases. (Class B fires generally involve materials that boil or bubble.)

Class C: Electrical: Energized electrical equipment as long as it is plugged in, it would be considered a class C fire. (Class C fires generally deal with electrical current.)

Class D: Metals: Potassium, sodium, aluminum, magnesium, unless one works in a laboratory or in an industry that uses these materials, it is unlikely that one has to deal with a Class D fire. It takes special extinguishing agents (Metal-X, foam) to fight such a fire.

Procedure for using fire extinguisher: Correct extinguisher must be used if it is an open fire, such as a large chemical spill on a lab bench. Operating a fire extinguisher correctly, involves pulling the pin, pointing the extinguisher at the base of the fire and squeezing the handle while moving the extinguisher back and forth. Care is taken so as not to spread the fire by getting the nozzle of the extinguisher too close to the material as the gas coming out of the fire extinguisher nozzle is under intense pressure. Cover the container with a piece of ceramic if it is a small fire, such as in a flask or beaker, cutting off the supply of oxygen to the fire and thus putting it out.

5. **Fire blankets:** If someone's clothes catch fire, wrapping quickly in the fire blanket will smother the fire. A fire blanket either completely surrounds a burning object or is placed over a burning object and sealed closely to a solid surface

around the fire. Whether the blanket is placed on top, or surrounding it, the job of the blanket is to cut off the oxygen supply to the fire, and put it out. The fire blanket will cover the fire and prevent oxygen from getting to it so that the fire cannot burn. What little oxygen is trapped under the fire blanket will quickly turn to carbon dioxide as the fire burns out. It is to be used only when the fire is not too large and is not a chemical fire that can burn without air. It should not to be thrown on a liquid fire or lab equipment, as it can spread, but it is very useful for individuals.

6. **Spill kits:** A spill kit should be accessible in every laboratory. The kit usually includes spill control pillows (which are commercially available), inert absorbents, such as vermiculite, clay, sand, neutralizing agents for acid spills such as sodium carbonate and sodium hydrogen carbonate, neutralizing agents for alkali spills such as sodium hydrogen sulfate and citric acid, large plastic scoops and other equipment such as brooms, pails, bags, and dust pans, appropriate personal protective equipment.

CHAPTER 2

Microscale Apparatus and Techniques

1. MICROSCALE GLASSWARES

Microscale chemistry is a laboratory-based, environmentally safe, pollution-preventive approach accomplished by using miniature glassware and significantly reduced amounts of chemicals. Microscale chemistry can be implemented without compromising educational standards or analytical rigor, and its techniques are amenable to industrial R&D applications.

Traditionally, experiments in organic chemistry are carried out on a macroscale level, employing chemicals of the order of 5–100 g, using glassware designed to contain between 25 and 500 ml liquids. For quantities of materials in the 0.005–0.5 g range, one employs different, technique called "microscale" which uses special glassware in order to carry out various standard organic laboratory operations.

I. TYPES OF GLASSWARE

a. **Ground-glass joints:** These are used to attach one piece of glass equipment to another with an air-tight seal (Fig. 2.1). The outer or female joint is conical with a slight taper and "ground" or rough on the inside. It slides the inner, or male joint which is conical and with the same taper and ground on the outside. Together they make a tight seal and join the two pieces. The joints are expensive because they are made to precise sizes and must fit perfectly. They come in standard sizes, called "standard taper", and are identified by two numbers, the first indicating the diameter of the joint and the second indicating the length of the tapered part. The first number is most important in matching the inner and outer joints. There are three sizes of standard taper (Ts) joints in microscale kit: 14/10, 7/10, and 5/5. Usually, these numbers are written on the glass part near the joint to facilitate matching of joint sizes.

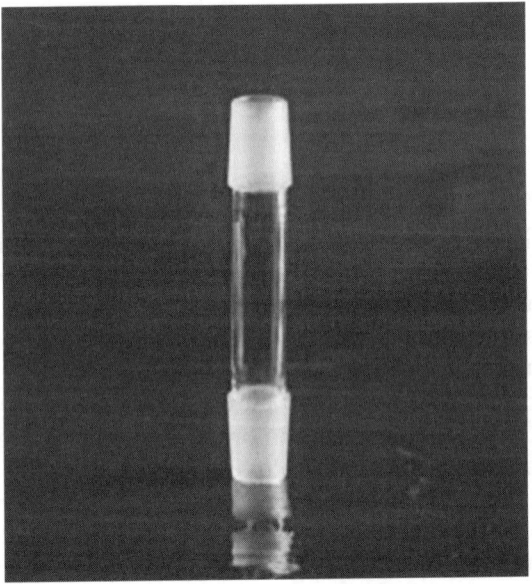

Fig. 2.1: Ground-glass joint

b. **Conical vials:** These take the place of large, round-bottom flasks used in the traditional laboratory (Fig. 2.2). Chemical reactions usually can be and are carried out in these vials. They can also be used for measuring and storing chemicals. Each one has an outer ground-glass joint and a threaded outer surface to allow attachment of other glassware. They are available in four sizes: 5.0, 3.0, 1.0, and 0.3 ml capacities. The two large sizes have a 14/10 outer joint, the 1 ml vial has a 7/10 joint, and the smallest vial has a 5/5 ground-glass joint at the top.

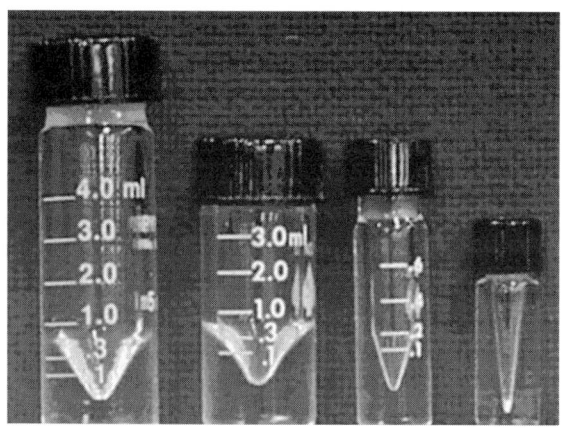

Fig. 2.2: Conical vials

c. **Air condensers:** These are glass tubes with an inner joint at the bottom and an outer joint at the top (Fig. 2.3). They are usually attached to a reaction vial (conical vial) and used to prevent vapors from escaping from a hot or boiling

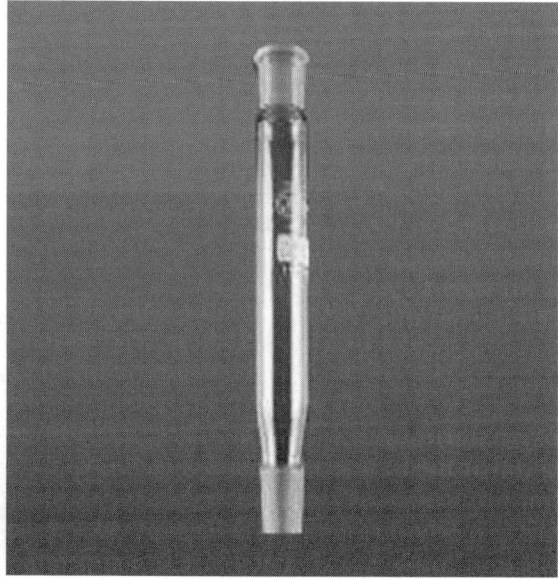

Fig. 2.3: Air condenser

reaction. The vapors come in contact with the cool inside surface of the tube and condense into the liquid phase, dripping down the inside of the tube and returning to the reaction mixture. Air which passes by the outer glass surface keeps the tube cool. The air condenser can also function as a simple mechanical extension to hold a conical vial in place in a cooling or heating bath. They come in two sizes which differ in the size of the ground-glass joints: the larger one has a 14/10 inner joint on the bottom and a smaller, 7/10 outer joint on top; the smaller one has 7/10 joints on top and bottom. The joint size must be matched with the joint size of the conical vial.

d. **Water-cooled or Jacketed condensers:** These serve the same purpose as the air condensers, except that cooling is made more efficient by circulating cold (tapwater or icewater) water through an outer glass jacket (Fig. 2.4). Water goes into the bottom connector and goes out from the top to prevent air trapping in the water jacket. For lower-boiling liquids, this additional cooling is necessary to prevent escape of vapors.

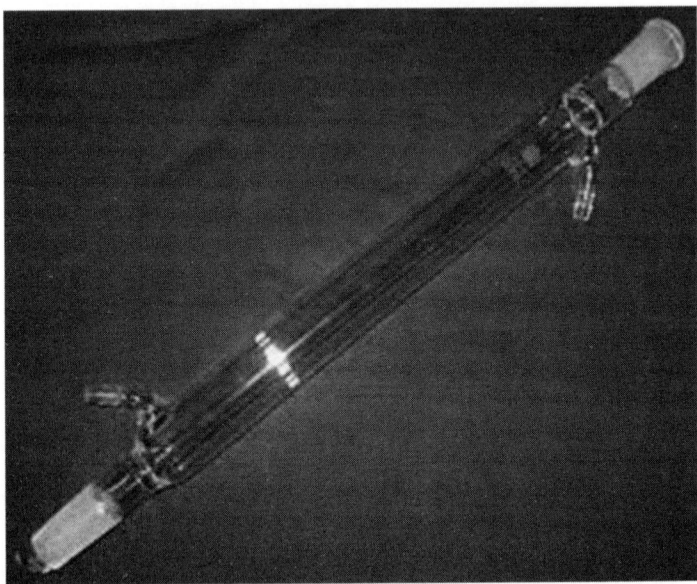

Fig. 2.4: Jacketed condenser

e. Claisen adaptor (head): This apparatus allows introducing chemical reagents (usually liquids) into a reaction mixture through the access hole at the top (Fig. 2.5). The chemicals can be added in the mixture without taking apart the entire apparatus. If a teflon liner and screw-cap are secured on the access hole, liquids can be introduced with a syringe without exposing the reaction mixture to the atmosphere. With a screw-cap and "O" ring, a thermometer can be introduced through the access hole.

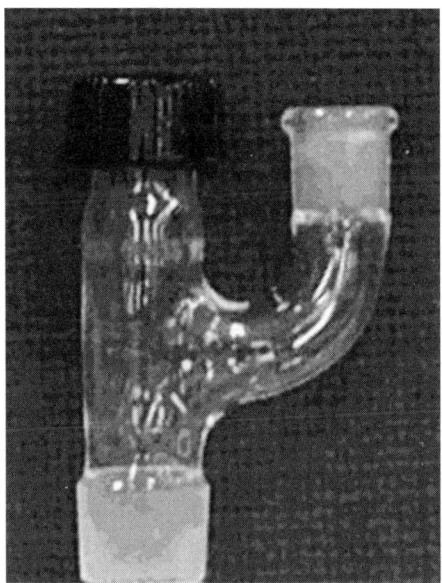

Fig. 2.5: Claisen adapter

f. Hickman distilling head: This versatile device replaces the traditional distilling unit, which is much larger and requires connecting and supporting a number of pieces of glassware (Fig. 2.6). The purpose of a still is to heat a liquid until is passes into the gas (vapor) phase, and then allow the vapor to cool and condense back into the liquid phase, with the condensed liquid trapped in a second container. The Hickman still functions like the air condenser in condensing vapors with the cool glass surface, but the liquid drips down the inside to be trapped in a small

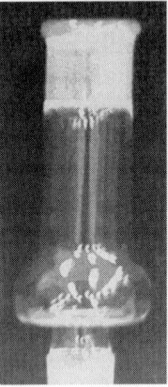

Fig. 2.6: Hickman distilling head

circular depression, or collar, in the lower part of the tube. The bottom joint is a 14/10 inner joint and the top joint is a 14/20 outer joint.

g. **Drying tube:** The drying tube attaches to the top of an apparatus with a 7/10 inner joint (Fig. 2.7). The tube is used to protect the reaction from moisture in the atmosphere while still allowing the passage of air to equalize pressure. To accomplish this, the tube is packed with appropriate quantity of moisture-absorbing solid (drying agent like silica gel, calcium chloride, etc.) surrounded by glass wool plugs on inner and outer side of it. This packing is done to prevent the drying agent from spilling out of the tube. It is important to remove the drying agent and clean the tube

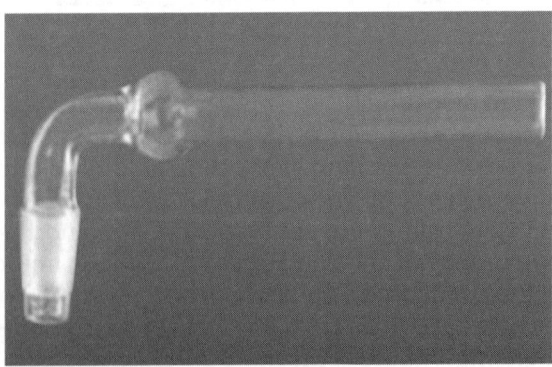

Fig. 2.7: Drying tube

after each use, since drying agents can harden and swell with time and become impossible to remove.

h. **Craig tube:** The Craig tube is used for small-scale recrystallization, which is a method for the purification of small quantities of solid compounds (Fig. 2.8). It has two parts: an outer **body**, which functions like a vial or test tube; and an inner **plunger**, which fits partly into the body and rests on a ground-glass surface. The ground-glass joint is not greased, so that liquids can leak through it but solids cannot pass.

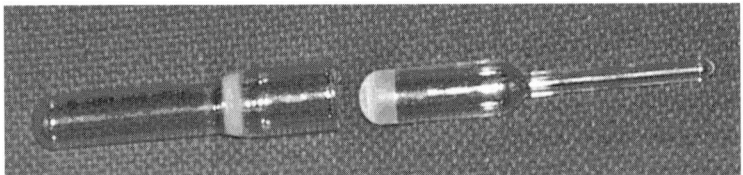

Fig. 2.8: Craig tube

i. **Capillary gas delivery tube:** This long tube has an inner 7/10 ground-glass joint on one end, four 90° bends, and a very small inside diameter (Fig. 2.9). It is placed on top of a reaction apparatus in which gas is generated, and the gas passes through the tube to be collected in an inverted tube at the other end. Gas collection is used to measure the quantity of gas produced in a reaction, or to prevent toxic gases from escaping to the atmosphere (by trapping them in water or some suitable solvent).

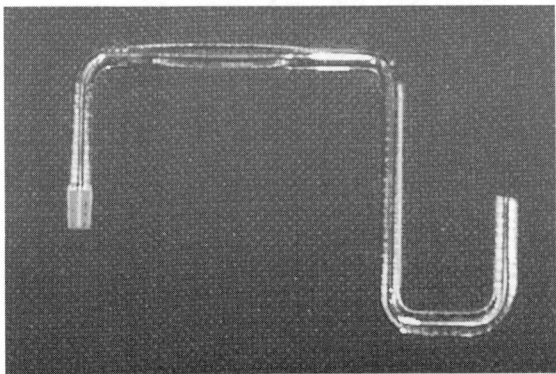

Fig. 2.9: Capillary gas delivery tube

j. **Pasteur pipette:** This pipette is used to transfer small quantities of liquids (Fig. 2.10). It is a glass tube tapered to a narrow point and fitted with a rubber bulb at the top. The combination of the Pasteur pipette and rubber bulb has also been referred to as a teat pipette. The constriction toward the tip of the Pasteur pipettes may be plugged with a bit of tissue paper or cotton wool to filter off solids from small amounts of liquids. Pasteur pipettes are also used for microscale distillations. The liquid to be distilled is placed into a small reaction tube along with a boiling chip and heated to reflux one-half to two-thirds of the way up the inside of the tube. After squeezing the bulb to expel air, a Pasteur pipette is inserted into the tube just below the level of the ring of refluxing liquid (into the vapor). The vapor is then drawn into the relatively cold pipette tip, causing it to condense and accumulate inside of the pipette. By this method, enough distillate can be collected to determine a boiling point, identify a distillate, or possibly prepare derivatives.

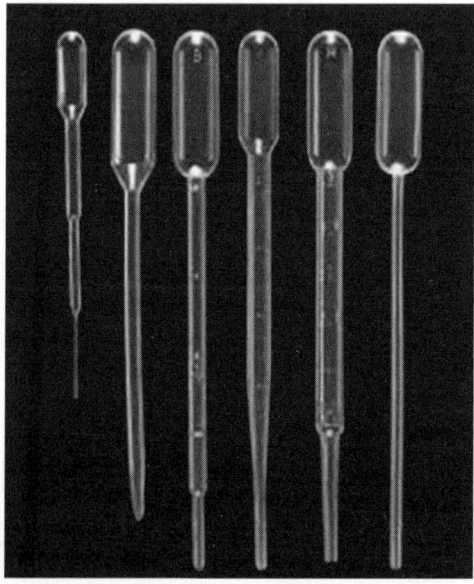

Fig. 2.10: Pasteur pipette

k. Micropipette: Micropipette is used to measure and transfer small volumes (< 1 ml) of liquids (Fig. 2.11). The scales on micropipettors are in microliters (1000 µl = 1 ml). It consists of plunger button, tip ejector button, volume adjustment dial, digital volume indicator, shaft and attachment point for a disposable tip).

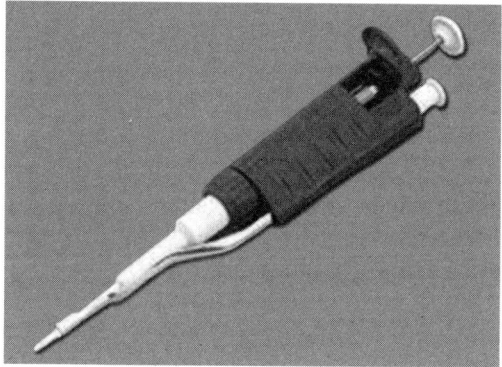

Fig. 2.11: Micropipette

l. Syringe: The syringe is really a medical device, but chemists use it regularly to measure and transfer small volumes of liquids (Fig. 2.12). It consists of three parts: the body, which is calibrated according to volume and has a metal fitting,

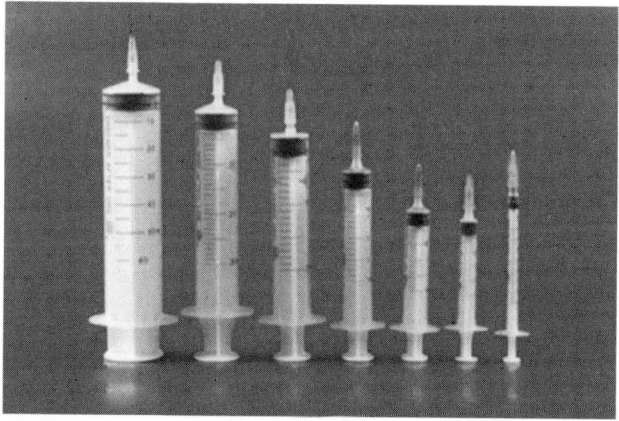

Fig. 2.12: Syringe

called a Luer-lock fitting; the plunger, which fits snugly into the body so that liquid cannot escape between the ground-glass outer surface of the plunger and the ground-glass inner surface of the body; and the needle, which is a hollow, pointed piece of stainless steel that connects to the syringe by way of the metal Luer-lock fitting.

m. **Magnetic stir vanes:** These are made of teflon with a small magnet embedded in the center. The magnet tends to align itself with a large magnet mounted just under the surface of the heater-stirrer. When the stirrer motor is started, the large magnet rotates and the spin vane, trying to stay aligned, rotates at the same time (Fig. 2.13). In this way, a heterogeneous reaction mixture can be continuously stirred without having to open the reaction vessel/apparatus and introduce a mechanical stirring device. The spin vane has a triangular shape that matches the triangular cross-section of the conical vials. It will not function unless it is placed in the vial with the point facing downward; it is a good idea to put it into the vial before adding chemicals or solvents. There are two sizes of spin vanes: the large one fits the two largest conical vials and the small one fits the 1 ml conical vial. They will not function in the wrong size vial, or in a beaker, vial, or flask which has a flat bottom. Spin vanes are

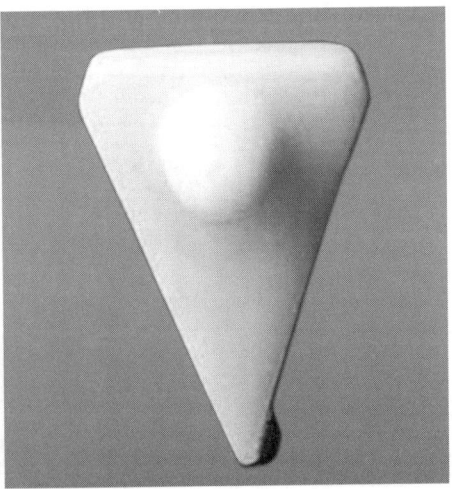

Fig. 2.13: Magnetic stir vane

very expensive and very easy to lose. These should be cleaned after each use and returned to the small vial that holds them.

n. **Magnetic stir bars:** These function on the same principle as the spin vane, but are designed for vessels that have a flat bottom (Fig. 2.14). They are just as expensive and easy to lose as the spin vanes.

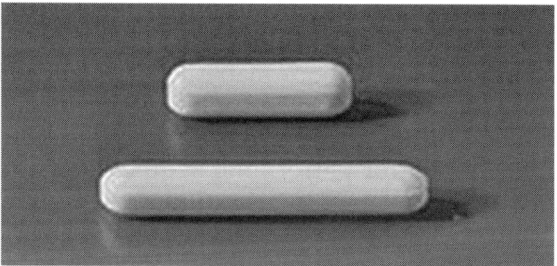

Fig. 2.14: Magnetic stir bars

o. **Microspatula:** This is one of the most useful devices in the microscale kit. The flat, long blade can be used to weigh solids, stir mixtures, remove "O" rings, scratch glass surfaces to induce crystallization, and generally poke at solutions to see what's going on (Fig. 2.15). It should be cleaned so that reactions and chemicals are not cross-contaminated.

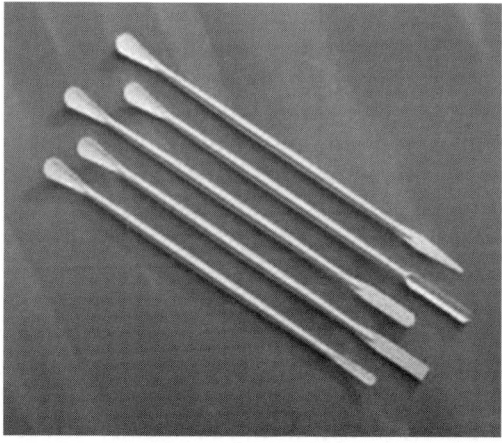

Fig. 2.15: Microspatula

II. STORAGE AND CARE

a. **Storage:** It is imperative that one should clean, dry and return all the glassware belonging in the common drawer/cabinet at the end of the laboratory period because other students in other sections are using the same glassware. A list of equipment belonging in the common drawer/cabinet and of that belonging in one's personal drawer should be provided at the beginning and should be kept in the personal drawer to keep track of what belongs where. These are expensive glassware and may not be available in plenty for each person. Hence, these should never be kept in the personal locker.

b. **Care and cleaning:** All the glassware must be clean and dry before it is used for performing synthesis. The nature of impurity will not be always known to us. If the used glassware is kept unattended and is left uncleaned, then the volatile matter will evaporate leaving behind the non-volatile residual impurities which might be very difficult to be removes when present in dried state. Moreover, in case of microscale glassware, one has to be additionally careful in handling it. Hence, to clean such glassware is extremely difficult. It must be kept in mind that there is no universal cleaning mixture recommended for any type of glassware. One should take into account the nature of substance to be removed. If the substance is acidic, strong basic solutions can also be used and vice versa is true for removing basic impurities. Also, one should be aware of the solvent in which the substance which is to be removed is soluble. In general, immediately after the reaction, wash the glassware with soap and then with water. Then, rinse it with a minimum amount of acetone to remove any organic compounds and dry it using the laboratory hot-air dryer. Never, ever put glassware that contains acetone in the microscale glassware kit. Acetone vapors will destroy the foam liners in the kit.

c. **Clean against clean and dry:** An experimental procedure calling for the use of clean glassware means that it should be washed with water and soap, followed by rinsing with water. This glassware is normally used when a water-containing reagent is used in the experiment (i.e. trace amounts on water on the glassware will not dramatically affect the results because an aqueous solution is being added to the glassware).

On the other hand, clean and dry glassware requires that the apparatus be washed and then dried; this is conveniently done by rinsing the apparatus with acetone after washing it and then drying it. Clean, dry equipment is used when it is essential to have no moisture present.

2. BASIC ORGANIC AND MICROSCALE TECHNIQUES

a. **Transferring and weighing liquids:** Never transfer a liquid to a container that is placed on the microbalance pan. Weigh the container, e.g. conical vial or sample vial), remove it from the balance, transfer the required volume of liquid, and reweigh the container to determine the actual weight used. In computing theoretical yield, use the actual weight of liquid that has been used. While using small containers and vials; ensure that these do not tip over, or get knocked over, by placing them in small beakers. When an experimental procedure requires the use of an "accurate" volume of liquid, e.g. 0.3 or 0.55 ml), use a syringe to measure the volume. This is usually required for measuring starting materials. Syringes color-coded with tape corresponding to color-coded reagent bottles are provided with the containers of liquid starting materials. Be certain to use the correct syringe with the correct reagent bottle and leave the syringe by the reagent bottles that are kept in the hoods. Never use the syringe from the kit for any reagent bottle in the hood! There is a risk of contamination of the entire reagent bottle because it is not known if the syringe is completely clean or not. When a procedure calls for the use of an approximate volume of liquid, e.g. about 1 or 2 ml), use a Pasteur pipette to measure the liquid. Approximate volumes are usually used in purification procedures (not as reactant) when it is not essential to use an exact volume. Pipettes hold their contents with the vacuum created when the pipette bulb is squeezed and then released to draw liquid into the pipette. If the pipette is tilted, vacuum may be lost and the liquid in the pipette may be lost and squirt out onto the bench, the lab notebook or even on the neighbor. A pipette tilted upside down will result in some of its contents running into and contaminating the inside of the pipette bulb. After using them, the pipettes can be washed and stored. Those that are too dirty to clean or are broken can be disposed of in the glass waste container. When larger volumes are required, (e.g. about 8 ml, etc.); graduated cylinders can be used. These will also be color-coded to their respective reagent bottles if used in the reagent hoods. To avoid having sample vials or conical vials tipped or knocked over, it is convenient to put them in the aluminum heating block, which is the microscale analog of a test tube rack for holding test tubes. However, do not leave the heating block in the personal drawer. Sample vials containing products may be placed in small beakers in the locker to avoid their falling over if it is necessary to keep them for further use.

b. **Transferring and weighing solids:** Never transfer a solid to a container that is kept on the microbalance pan. While weighing a solid starting material, place a piece of weighing paper (butter paper) on the balance pan. Weighing paper is good for transferring solids because they do not stick to the paper. Carefully transfer the solid on the paper with the help of a clean microspatula until the desired weight is obtained. Then, carefully transfer the solid directly to a conical reaction vial or to a clean dry, small sample vial if the solid is to be added to a reaction mixture (e.g. to a conical vial) in small quantities. It is highly unlikely that one is able to weigh the exact weight of solid required for a reaction. In determining the weight of a solid product, weigh the clean, dry sample vial, remove it from the balance, transfer solid to it and reweigh the container to determine the actual weight of the product (weighing by difference). To avoid having sample vials or conical vials tipped or knocked over, it is convenient to put them in the aluminum heating block.

c. **Addition to reaction mixtures (solids, liquids and gases) Addition of solids:** Solid compounds and reagents are usually added to the reaction flask by removing the stopper. In case, when the solid is needed to be added to a boiling reaction mixture, then the heating is stopped, reaction mixture is allowed to cool and the solid is added to it. If the solid is required to be added without opening the reaction flask to maintain inert atmospheric conditions, Gooch tubing is used. This is a thin flexible rubber tubing which is fitted over the neck of reaction mixture in which addition is to be done and over the neck of flask from which solid is to be added. However, this method cannot be used in case when addition causes evolution of heat and gases.

Addition of liquids: Reactions involving addition of liquids in a controlled manner are carried out in two-necked or three-necked round bottom flasks equipped with an addition funnel. This addition funnel resembles a separating funnel with standard-taper joint at the outlet. It is used with the stopper opened while addition of liquid or solution is being done. For inert atmospheric operations, pressure-equilibrated addition funnels can be used which are stoppered. Stopcocks with teflon sealing are preferred over those which are greased because the grease can be leached by organic liquids which may contaminate the reaction mixture.

Addition of gases: A gas may be added to a reaction mixture through a glass tube or hypodermic needle that dips below the surface of the liquid. It is desirable to direct the gas to the bottom surface of the reaction mixture if the gas is highly soluble or highly reactive. If the gas reacts to form a precipitate, care should be taken to prevent clogging of the inlet tube.

d. **Stirring and mixing:** Magnetic stirrer is the most commonly used equipment for efficient stirring and mixing. It consists of a variable speed motor which spins a magnet. The reaction mixture along with the magnetic bar or rod is placed on the base of magnetic stirrer. Such stirrer is very useful for stirring mixtures that are not too viscous or do not contain heavy precipitates. For the reaction mixtures that are difficult to stir, direct drive mechanical stirrers are employed.

e. **Drying methods**

Drying of solids: The solid compounds can be dried by allowing them to stand in an evaporating dish, beaker, petri dish. Rigorous drying can be done by making use of desiccators. In this method, drying agents such as silica gel, phosphorus pentoxide, calcium sulphate, magnesium perchlorate is placed in the bottom of the dessicator and the solid compound is placed in an open container that is rested on the dessicant. Greater efficiency can be achieved by evacuation of the dessicator. Large amount of solids can be dried by placing them in vacuum ovens.

Drying of liquids and solutions: Liquids and solutions containing small amounts of water can be dried by allowing them to stand in contact with drying agent for a suitable period of time followed by decantation or filtration. Some common drying agents used are sodium sulphate, calcium sulphate, calcium chloride, potassium carbonate, magnesium sulphate and a few more. These dried liquids can be kept free from water by storing over molecular sieves. These sieves are synthetic zeolites possessing cavities of uniform size which incorporate small molecules. Sieves of 3 and 4°A are capable of trapping water molecules. Small quantities of solvents or liquid reagents can be dried by passing through a short column of activated alumina.

Drying of gases: Water vapours can be removed from a gas by passing the gas through a drying tower containing pellets of a desiccant or through a gas wash bottle containing concentrated sulphuric acid.

f. **Removal of solvents:** This is particular useful when we have to obtain a desired product from a reaction mixture, a chromatographic fraction, an extract or from mother liquor after recrystallization. These solvents can be removed by simple or fractional distillation under at atmospheric pressure or under reduced pressure but with due consideration given to the stability and volatility of the desired product. Care must be taken to prevent the decomposition of product due to overheating. The removal of volatile solvents from the product can be efficiently done by using rotary evaporator. The flask is filled to half or less than half of its capacity and is immersed in water bath, pressure of the system is reduced by the aspirator and flask is rotated. The rotation prevents bumping and increases the surface area for wetting the warmed or hot walls of the flask from which evaporation becomes rapid.

Some commonly used organic solvents

Name of solvent	Chemical formula	Boiling point (°C)	Density (gm/c.c)	Flammability	Miscibility with water	Health hazard
Acetone	$CH_3-CO-CH_3$	56	0.78	Highly flammable	Miscible	Low
Methanol	CH_3OH	65	0.79	Flammable	Miscible	Low
Ethanol (Absolute)	$CH_3\ CH_2OH$	78.5	0.78	Flammable	Miscible	Low
Dimethyl formamide	$HCON(CH_3)_2$	153	0.94	Flammable	Miscible	High
Dimethyl sulphoxide	$CH_3-SO-CH_3$	189	1.1	Flammable	Miscible	Low
Chloroform	$CHCl_3$	61	1.48	Nonflammable	Immiscible	High
Ethyl acetate	$CH_3-COO-C_2H_5$	77	0.92	Flammable	Immiscible	Low
Isopropyl alcohol	$CH_3-CHOH-CH_3$	82	0.78	Flammable	Miscible	Low
Tetrahydro furan	⬠	66	0.9	Flammable	Miscible	Moderate
Dichloromethane	CH_2Cl_2	40	1.42	Poorly flammable	Immiscible	Low
Benzene	C_6H_6	80	0.87	Flammable	Immiscible	High
Diethyl Ether	$C_2H_5-O-C_2H_5$	35	0.70	Highly flammable	Immiscible	Low
Hexane	$CH_3\ (CH_2)_4\ CH_3$	69	0.65	Flammable	Immiscible	Low
Pentane	$CH_3\ (CH_2)_3\ CH_3$	36	0.62	Highly flammable	Immiscible	Low
Carbon disulphide	CS_2	46	1.2	Highly flammable	Immiscible	High
Toluene	$C_6H_5\ CH_3$	111	0.86	Flammable	Immiscible	Moderate
Acetonitrile	CH_3CN	82	0.78	Flammable	Miscible	Moderate
Carbon tetrachloride	CCl_4	77	1.58	Nonflammable	Immiscible	High

g. Melting point determination:

Definition: The melting point of a substance is defined as the temperature at which the material changes from a solid to a liquid state at atmospheric pressure.

Melting point determination is considered to be a simple and fast method used in diverse areas of chemistry to get a first impression of the purity of a substance. This is because even small quantities of impurities cause depression of the melting point and increases the melting point range. This test is a fast and cost-effective technique and is still an important method for gauging purity of organic and pharmaceutical compounds. It is one of the oldest identification test applied for many organic substances. The melting point is easy to measure, tabulate and classify. Exhaustive literature survey is available in scientific books, which enlists the standard melting point of nearly all the organic compounds and drugs.

Sample preparation and requirements: Careless preparation of a sample is the leading cause of incorrect and irreproducible results in melting point determinations. The accuracy and reproducibility of melting point measurement is highly dependent upon the way in which sample is prepared and the visual observation of changes in the sample can also lead to unreliable results. A clear, sharply defined melting point indicates that the sample has a high state of purity.

Any substance being loaded into a melting point capillary must be fully dried, homogeneous and in powdered form. The basic requirement for a good melting point determination is that the sample should be in a fine powder form. This helps in transferring the heat in the sample more efficiently and in a reproducible way. Samples which are crystalline, coarse and non-homogeneous must be crushed into a fine powder [usually in a mortar] and then subjected to melting point determination. If the sample is hygroscopic in nature, or sublimates at high temperatures, the open end of the capillary tube must be sealed by heating. Hygroscopic samples must be stored in a desiccator all the time. This is especially critical in humid environments or rainy days. It is a good practice to wipe the outside surface of the capillary tube with a clean cloth or tissue paper before subjecting it to melting point determination. It is also recommended that the same batch of capillaries should be used for various determinations of the same samples to assure the repeatability of results as all capillaries do not have same dimensions.

Filling of capillary: The melting point sample is held inside thin walled capillary melting point tube. This tube needs to be sealed at one end. Pre-sealed tubes if available in the laboratory or an open capillary can be sealed by inserting the tip into a Bunsen flame near the base of the flame for sealing it. For filling the capillary tube with a sample, the open end of the capillary is pressed gently into the substance kept on a watch glass or weighing paper several times. To transfer the crystals from the open end to the bottom of the tube, tap the bottom gently on the bench top or scratch the top edge of the tube on a small file or a coin with a rough edge without breaking the capillary tube. The tube should be densely packed with the substance. In addition to tight packing, maintaining a fixed level in the fill is also a very important requirement. Taller samples take extra heat to completely melt and usually display larger melting ranges than their shorter counterparts. A sample height between 2.0 and 3.0 mm is recommended for optimum results and reproducibility.

Methods for determination of melting point:

1. **Using Thiele's tube:** The Thiele's tube is a glass tube designed to contain heating oil and a thermometer to which a capillary tube containing the sample is attached. The shape of the Thiele's tube allows for formation of convection currents in the oil when it is heated. These currents maintain a fairly uniform temperature distribution throughout the oil in the tube. The side arm of the tube is designed to generate these convection currents and thus transfer the heat from the flame evenly and rapidly throughout the heating oil. The sample, packed in a capillary tube, is attached to the thermometer and held by means of a rubber band or a small slice of rubber tubing. It is important that this rubber band be above the level of the oil thus allowing for expansion of the oil

allows the capillary tube to fall into the oil. The Thiele's tube is usually heated using a Bunsen burner as shown in Fig. 2.16. During heating, the rate of rise of temperature should be carefully controlled. One should hold the burner by its base and using a small, gentle flame, move the burner slowly back and forth along the bottom of the side arm of the Thiele's tube. If the heating rate is too fast, the burner is removed for a few seconds before resuming the heating process. The rate of heating should be slow near the melting point (about 1–2°C per minute) to ensure that the rate of temperature increase is not faster than the ability of the heat to be transferred to the sample being observed.

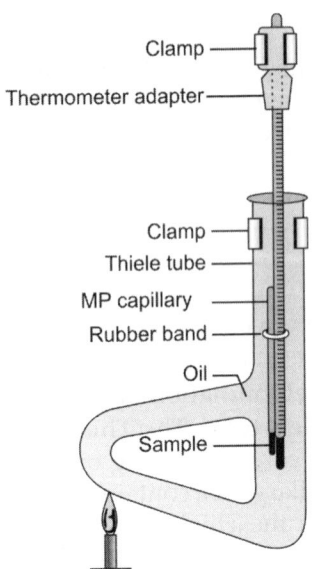

Fig. 2.16: Melting point determination by Thiele's tube

2. **Using melting point apparatus:** A melting point apparatus consists of a slot to insert thermometer and wells to insert capillary tubes containing samples located on the front of the thermometer tube. Usually, there are wells for inserting three capillaries. The power switch is turned "on" and the heating control knob is adjusted in

order to set the power level to obtain the desired heating rate. The sample can be observed through the lens on the front of the apparatus. A slow heating rate is kept when the melting starts in order to get an accurate measurement. The temperature on the thermometer is recorded when the sample starts to melt and again recorded when the sample has melted to get the melting point range. Once the sample has completely melted, the power is turned "off" and the capillary is removed and disposed in the container maintained for this purpose.

h. **Boiling point determination**

Definition: The boiling point of a liquid substance is defined as the temperature at which the vapor pressure of a liquid is equal to the atmospheric pressure on the liquid.

Like melting point, determination of boiling point is also considered to serve as a characteristic physical property for that liquid compound. If the boiling point is higher the liquid will be less volatile and vice versa. In general, compounds with ionic bonds raise the melting points and boiling points, if they do not decompose before reaching such high temperatures. Also, higher boiling point is associated with compounds containing more covalently bonds and greater molecular mass. Sometimes, when the molecular size becomes that of a macromolecule, polymer, or otherwise very large, the compound often decomposes at high temperature before the boiling point is reached. Boiling point is also raised by increase in the polarity of a molecule.

The presence of non-volatile impurities such as salts decreases the compound's volatility and thus raises the boiling point. This effect is called boiling point elevation. As a common example, salt water boils at a higher temperature than pure water.

Methods for determination of boiling point:

1. **Using Thiele's tube:** If only small amounts of liquid material are available for boiling point determination, then a micro boiling point apparatus based on a Thiele's tube should be used. This tube contains heating oil and a thermometer to which a micro test tube containing the

boiling point sample is attached. The Thiele's tube should not be clamped too tightly otherwise it might crack as it expands on heating. The sample liquid is introduced by Pasteur pipette into a micro test tube. This test tube should not be of more than 0.5 ml capacity with a depth of about 10 mm, and a piece of melting point capillary tubing (sealed at one end) is dropped in with the open end down. The micro test tube assembly is then attached to a thermometer with a rubber band or a thin slice of rubber tubing. The whole unit is then placed in the Thiele's tube.

The placement of the test tube/thermometer unit in the Thiele's tube is important. The micro test tube should be on the same side of the Thiele's tube. Neither the test tube nor the thermometer bulb should be touching the glass walls of the Thiele's tube. The base of the micro test tube should be just below the joint to the upper part. The rubber band should be placed well above the level of the oil in the Thiele's tube. The oil level should be just above the top of the top elbow joint. When positioning the rubber band, one should bear in mind that the oil will expand when it is heated.

Once the set up has been complete, the lower part of the side arm of the Thiele's tube is carefully heated with a small flame from the Bunsen burner moving the flame back and forth along the arm. During the heating, there is an initial stream of bubbles from the capillary tube as air is expelled and then, a little later, a rapid and continuous stream of bubbles emerges from the inverted capillary tube. At this point stop heating. Soon the stream of bubbles will slow down and stop. When they stop, the liquid sample will be drawn up into the capillary tube. The moment liquid enters the capillary corresponds to the boiling point of the liquid, and the temperature should be recorded.

During the initial heating, the air trapped in the capillary tube expands and leaves the tube and vapor from the liquid also enters the tube. There is always vapor in equilibrium with a heated liquid. This gives rise to the initial stream of bubbles. When the temperature reaches the boiling point, the vapor pressure inside the capillary tube equals the atmospheric pressure. As the temperature rises just above the boiling point then the vapor will start to escape. Once the heating is stopped, the only vapor left in the capillary comes from the heated liquid which seals its open end. As the liquid cools, its vapor pressure will decrease and when the vapor pressure drops just below atmospheric pressure, the liquid will be drawn [sucked] into the capillary tube.

2. **By heating:** When relatively large amounts of liquid are available, boiling points can be determined using a distillation method or by simply heating the liquid in a test tube in which a thermometer is inserted so that it does not touch the walls of the test tube as depicted in Fig. 2.17. When the liquid is boiling freely, then that is the boiling temperature. Only the lower portion of the test tube must be heated. A sand bath may also be used, if preferred. Direct flame is not used on the test tube. A cork with a small slit cut in it may be used instead of the thermometer adapter and syringe needle as shown in the figure. Ensure that there is a way for vapor to escape. After the se-up is complete, drop a fresh boiling chip into the test tube. Then add the liquid whose boiling point is

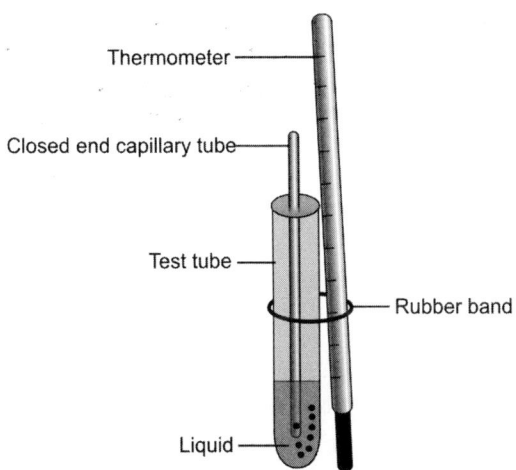

Fig. 2.17: Boiling point determination

to be determined. Insert the thermometer carefully so as not to break it. The thermometer should not touch the glass test tube and there should be enough liquid to cover the thermometer bulb a short way up the stem. The boiling temperature is the steady temperature observed usually for about one minute, when refluxing occurs over the lower part of the thermometer and not all the way up to the top of the test tube.

a. General methods of heating

i. Heating using sand bath: A commonly used means of heating chemical reactions on a small scale is to use a sand bath. The sand bath consists of a petri dish or a small crystallizing dish (thermostable) that has been filled to a depth of about 1 cm with sand. The sand bath is also heated by placing it on a hot plate. The temperature of the sand bath may be monitored by clamping a thermometer in position so that the bulb of the thermometer is buried in the sand. The high sides of the crystallizing dish act to protect the apparatus from air drafts and hence, the dish also operates somewhat as a hot-air bath. More uniform heating can be made by covering the crystallizing dish with aluminum foil. A sand bath, with thermometer, is shown in Fig. 2.18. It is recommended that an aluminum block,

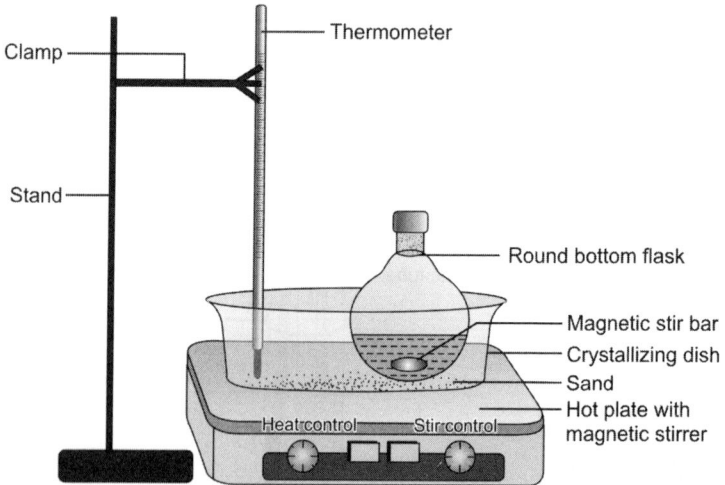

Fig. 2.18: Hot plate-magnetic stirrer with sand bath and reaction flask

rather than a sand bath, be used as a heating source whenever possible. The aluminum block can be heated and cooled quickly, it is indestructible, and there are no problems with spillage of sand.

j. **Reflux using sand bath:** Refluxing refers to boiling a solution and condensing the vapors in a manner that allows return of the condensate to the reaction flask. The purpose of refluxing in organic synthesis is to maintain reaction mixture at a constant and desired temperature. Boiling chips are added to the refluxing mixture to prevent bumping and promote smooth boiling.

In microscale reactions, two basic types of reflux condensers are utilized: the aircooled condenser or air condenser as shown in Fig. 2.19, and the water-jacketed condenser as shown in Fig. 2.20. Air condenser is adequate for those reactions which involve higher boiling solvents with no water passing through the condenser. A water-jacketed condenser is used for cases where the solvent is very volatile or low boiling or where the ambient air temperature is very high. A spin vane might also be included for magnetic stirring of the reaction mixture. Note that the apparatus should be clamped at the condenser

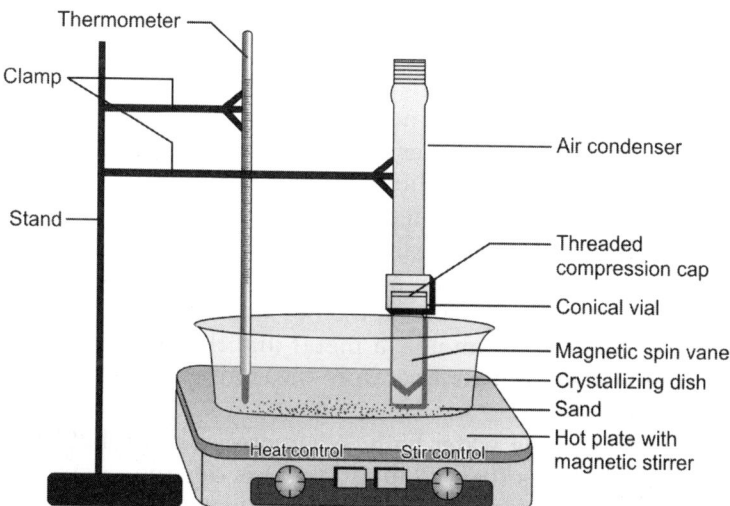

Fig. 2.19: Air condenser with conical vial; for heating and magnetic stirring

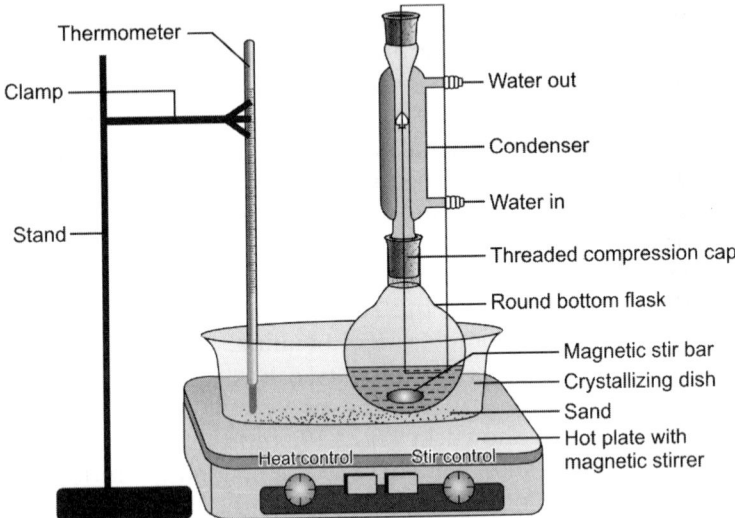

Fig. 2.20: Water-jacketed condenser with round bottom flask; for heating and magnetic stirring

rather than at the flask, as one would do for a macroscale experiment using conventional ground-glass joint glass-ware. The apparatus can be clamped in this way because of the screw-cap connection between the condenser and reaction vial, which prevents the connection from falling apart. Heating is provided by a sand bath atop a magnetic stirrer/heater. A thermometer is clamped in contact with the sand so as to allow monitoring of the bath temperature. It is important to have enough sand to ensure good thermal contact with the reaction vial, but not so much that it is difficult to see the contents.

Caution: A mercury thermometer should not be used in direct contact with an aluminum block. If it breaks, the mercury will vaporize on the hot surface. Instead, a non-mercury thermometer, a metal dial thermometer, or a digital electronic temperature-measuring device must be used.

k. **Heating using water bath:** When precise control at lower temperatures (below about 80°C) is desired, a suitable alternative is to use a water bath. The water bath consists of a vessel filled with water to the required depth. The hot plate is used to heat the water bath to the desired temperature. The water in the water bath will evaporate during heating. It is essential to maintain the water level in the water bath nearly constant to prevent charring or burning of reaction mixture.

1. **Distillation:** The key to successful microscale distillations is in avoiding long distillation paths, since this is the main factor leading to loss of material during distillation. Short-path microscale distillations are carried out using Hickman distillation head as the receiving device for the distilled liquid as shown in Fig. 2.21. The complete apparatus consists of a flask or vial containing the liquid and a magnetic spin vane or boiling stone/chip, attached to the bottom joint of the Hickman head. If required, a condenser

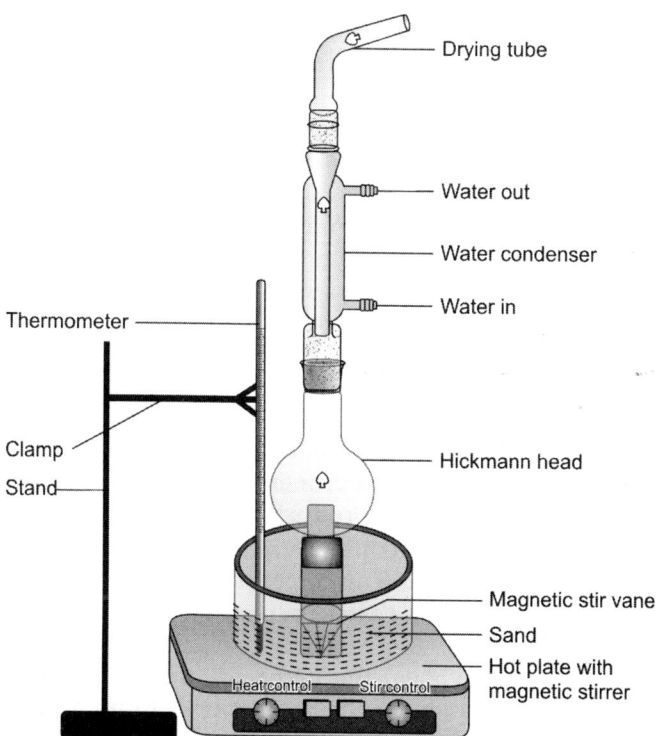

Fig. 2.21: Microscale distillation using the Hickman distillation head

can be attached to the top joint. A thermometer is suspended down the middle in order to record the distilling temperature, with the bottom of the thermometer in the lower part of the Hickman head just below the circular well. The vapors of the heated liquid rise upward and are cooled and condensed on either the inside walls of the Hickman head or on the walls of the condenser. As the liquid drains downward, it collects in the circular well at the bottom of the still. The well can contain as much as 2 ml of liquid. Collection of fractions is easiest with the ported Hickman head; the port is opened and the liquid in the well-removed with a Pasteur pipette. With the unported head, the liquid is drawn out from the top with a Pasteur pipette. If a condenser or internal thermometer is used, the distilling apparatus must be partially disassembled in order to do this. In some stills, the inner diameter of the head is so small that it is difficult to reach in at an angle with the pipette and make contact with the liquid. This problem may be remedied by bending the tip of the pipette slightly in a flame or by using a flexible plastic pipette. Once removed, the liquid is transferred to a small vial and capped with a teflon-sealed cap.

m. **Extraction:** Many experimental procedures involving organic liquids require either washing the organic layer or extracting a desired compound from a reaction mixture. A useful and easy way to perform extractions or washings is to use a conical vial or a large sample vial, as described below. Depending on the experiment, the lower layer or the upper layer contains the desired compound and the experimental procedure will indicate which layer to keep. To avoid repeating an experiment, it is advisable to save all layers until the desired product is obtained.

1. **Extraction using conical vials:** Mix the organic and aqueous layers in a 5 ml conical vial by drawing some of the mixture into a Pasteur pipette and expelling it back into the vial. Repeat this process several times. Alternatively, seal the vial with a cap containing a septum, and shake the vial gently. Remember that pressure can build up inside the vial, so make sure the vial is upright and carefully remove the cap of a vial that

has been shaken. When mixing is complete, allow the layers to separate, and use a Pasteur pipette to remove the lower layer first. Squeeze the bulb first, lower the pipette into the solution, through the top layer and into the bottom layer and slowly release the bulb to allow the pipette to "suck up" the liquid from the lower layer. Repeat this process, as necessary, until the entire bottom layer is removed. This process takes advantage of the taper of the conical vial and allows for better and more complete separation of the layers. Be careful not to draw the upper layer into the pipette.

2. **Extraction using large sample vials:** Mix the organic and aqueous layers in a large sample vial and cap it tightly. Make sure the cap has a plastic insert in it. The top rim of the sample vial should be free of cracks to avoid leakage. Shake the vial gently, and release the pressure by opening and retightening the cap periodically. Allow the layers to separate. Hold the vial at an angle and using a Pasteur pipette, remove the lower layer, using the technique described above for the conical vials.

n. **Recrystallization:** Crystallization is the deposition of crystals from a solution of given substance. During this process, several molecules of similar structure get attached to each other because these fit in the crystal lattice more properly than with other molecules of different structures. Recrystallization depends upon the difference in solubility of the substance in a hot and a cold solvent. In order to recover the starting material, it is desirable to have solubility of the substance to be high in hot solvent and low in cold solvent. Solvent having relatively low boiling point is preferred to carry out recrystallization as it can be easily removed by evaporation. If the structure of the substance is known and contains polar functional groups, then it should be soluble in polar solvent and vice versa is also true.

Recrystallization on microscale basis can be carried out using a conical reaction vial and conventional vacuum filtration to collect the crystals on a small filter paper. In recrystallization with a conical reaction vial, the conical vial simply takes the place of the Erlenmeyer flask used for

Some common solvents used for recrystallization (in the order of decreasing polarity)	
Sr. No. Solvent	*Polarity Index*
1. Water	10.3
2. Dimethyl sulphoxide (DMSO)	7.2
3. Methanol	6.6
4. Dimethyl formamide (DMF)	6.4
5. Acetonitrile	5.9
6. Ethanol	5.2
7. Acetone	5.1
8. Chloroform	4.4
9. Ethyl acetate	4.4
10. Isopropyl alcohol	4.3
11. Dichloromethane	3.4
12. Diethyl ether	2.8
13. Benzene	2.7
14. Toluene	2.4
15. Carbon tetrachloride	1.6
16. Hexane	0.1

macroscale recrystallization. The isolation of the crystals can be done in a number of ways as follows:

i. Once crystallization is complete, the mother liquor and crystals are vacuum-filtered through a small Hirsch funnel. Most commonly, the material is transferred to the funnel by pouring, using a microspatula to help transfer the crystals from the vial to the filter. In cases where the crystals are fairly small and fluffy, it may be more convenient to draw the entire mixture of crystals and mother liquor into a Pasteur pipette and transfer them to the Hirsch funnel.

ii. If the crystals adhere to the side of the flask, then filtration is unnecessary. Simply use a filter-tip pipette to remove the mother liquor and transfer it to another flask. Fresh, cold solvent is added to wash the crystals, and this is then removed with the pipette in the same way. The crystals are then dried using a very light stream of air or nitrogen, but care must be taken to ensure that the stream is light enough that the crystals don't get blown out of the vial.

Some worked-out examples of crystallization:

1. **Microscale recrystallization of acetylsalicylic acid from water:** Calculate the required minimum volume of hot water to dissolve 60 mg of acetylsalicylic acid (aspirin). The solubility of acetylsalicylic acid in water at 25°C is 1.0 g/300 ml and at 37°C is 1.0 g/100 ml. It will hydrolyze in boiling water, so do not heat the recrystallization solution for long. Heat until the bubbles begin to form. Use the aspirin solubility at 37°C for hot solubility calculation and reduce the solvent volume by 1/3 to 1/2 (guessing at the higher solubility of aspirin in 100°C water). Place 60 mg of acetylsalicylic acid in a reaction tube and add the required minimum volume of water calculated above. Add a boiling stick and start gently heating on the sand bath. As water begins to boil, add water dropwise until the sample just dissolves. Add 1 more drop of water. Remove the solution from heat and place in the test tube holder to cool to room temperature undisturbed. If crystals do not form upon cooling, scratch the side of the reaction tube with a glass rod. If crystals still do not form, ask for help on the next steps to take. Once crystals have formed, place the reaction tube in an ice bath and allow crystallization to complete. Once the reaction tube is ice-cold and no further crystallization occurs, proceed with the following isolation steps.

   a. Place the tip of Pasteur pipette firmly on the bottom of the reaction tube (not so firmly as to break the pipette stem).

   b. Draw the solvent away from the crystals leaving as many crystals as possible. There should be very few crystals in pipette stem.

   c. If too many crystals enter the pipette, use the vacuum filtration apparatus with the Hirsch funnel to isolate the crystals. The Hirsch funnel and vacuum is also a good way to pre-dry the crystals.

d. Complete the drying of crystals that are in the reaction tube by attaching it to an aspirator apparatus and gently heat over a steam bath while the crystals in the pipette are undergoing vacuum drying.

e. All residual solvent must be removed before using the aspirator drying technique.

f. Remove the crystals from the reaction tube by scraping with a spatula and complete the drying in the drying oven, if necessary.

g. Weigh the dry crystals. Take the melting point of dry crystals and of the crude product.

2. **Microscale recrystallization of naphthalene from 80% methanol (solvent):** Recrystallize naphthalene (40 mg) from the solvent. Place 40 mg of naphthalene in a reaction tube and add few drops of solvent, just enough to cover the crystals. Add a boiling stick and heat gently over the steam bath. Add solvent dropwise as the mixture comes to boiling. Methanol is relatively low boiling and will evaporate readily if heated strongly, hence heat gently. Once all of the crystals have dissolved, add one more drop of solvent and remove the reaction tube from the steam bath. Place the reaction tube in a test tube stand and allow to cool to room temperature undisturbed. Follow the normal procedure if crystal growth does not occur. Once crystals are observed, place the reaction tube in an ice bath and allow crystallization to complete. Remove the solvent by pipette as previously described. Scrape the crystals onto filter paper and allow them to air dry for 10–15 minutes. Do not heat the crystals as naphthalene will sublime. Do not dry the crystals in the drying oven for the same reason. Do not air dry naphthalene for prolonged periods (days) or product may be lost due to sublimation. It can be stored in a screw top vial to prevent loss. Once the naphthalene is dry, weigh the crystals and determine the melting point.

3. **Microscale recrystallization of benzoin from 95% ethanol (solvent):** Place about 250 mg of benzoin in a 25 ml Erlenmeyer flask. Add a boiling chip, stirring rod or if a magnetic stirring hot plate is used, a small magnetic bar. Add enough preheated solvent to cover the crystals and then heat on a

sand bath. When the mixture is at a low boil, add dropwise (Pasteur pipette) small amounts of the solvent just to the point where all the benzoin goes into solution. The solution may be colored and that it may have some insoluble impurities still present. Cool the solution somewhat and add carefully about 1–5 mg of activated charcoal to adsorb the colored impurities. If powdered charcoal is used, one must be careful during the addition, since frothing may occur. Heat the solution to boiling once again with stirring. Filter the hot solution (Caution! hold the flask with tongs or use a towel) into another 25 ml Erlenmeyer flask using a short stem funnel or better a stemless one . Pre-heat the funnel with hot solvent. During the filtration, crystals may appear in the funnel due to the cooling or evaporation of the solution. This can often be avoided by pre-heating the funnel or by heating the solution in the receiving flask during the process so that warm vapors envelop the funnel. Once the filtration is complete, add a small amount of hot solvent to the original flask and pass this through the filter. Concentrate the warm filtrate by heating the flask using stir bar on a sand bath in the hood to the point where the original volume of solvent used remains. Allow the flask to cool to room temperature. If crystals do not appear, concentrate the solution further and recool. At this point it may be necessary to add a seed crystal or to scratch the walls of the flask with a glass rod (this is most successful if carried out at the interface of the solution surface with the flask) to induce crystallization. Finally, place the flask and contents in an ice–water bath for 10–15 minutes to complete crystallization. Recover the crystals by suction filtration using a Hirsch funnel. Wash the crystals carefully with a small amount of cold solvent. To do this operation, vent the vacuum pump and add a small amount of ice-cold solvent over the crystals. Drain off the wash by closing the vent and repeat once or twice more, if necessary. Continue to apply reduced pressure to the filter plate to aid in drying the crystals. Determine the melting point and compare it to the literature value. Calculate the percent recovery.

4. **Microscale recrystallization of an unknown:** Measure the solubility properties of the unknown using 10 mg sample

and water, ethanol, and methanol. Determine the appropriate solvent to recrystallize the unknown. Keep in mind that the unknown will have insoluble impurities. Not all material will dissolve. Look for differently colored material that does not dissolve. This is insoluble impurity and does not affect the decision in selection of the appropriate solvent for recrystallization. Accurately weigh approximately 1.0 g of impure unknown. Place it in a 50–125 ml Erlenmeyer flask and add the selected solvent dropwise until the crystals are just covered with solvent. Begin heating using a hot plate until the solvent boils gently. Add solvent dropwise until the crystals dissolve. Insoluble impurties will not dissolve. These impurities may have a different color or different crystal type than the unknown which makes up the bulk of the crystals. Once the crystals have just dissolved, add 5% more solvent. Remove the insoluble impurities. Filter the hot solution by gravity filtration using fluted filter paper. The plastic funnel should be heated on the steam bath just before use. Hot solvent should be available at this time. The receiving Erlenmeyer flask should also be heated either on the steam bath or hot plate (add a small amount of solvent to the flask if using a hot plate). Place the fluted filter paper into the hot funnel. Place the filter paper and funnel onto the heated receiving Erlenmeyer flask which should be placed on a ceramic disk just prior to use. Pour the hot recrystallization mixture as quickly as possible into the fluted filter paper. Use a clamp (burette or universal), paper towel ring, or other suitable means to avoid burning the fingers as the hot solution is poured. Allow the solution to drain through the paper. Pour a small volume (no more than 1–2 ml) of hot solvent through the paper to dissolve any crystals that have precipitated on the paper or on the funnel sides. Place the flask containing hot solution in ice bath for 10–15 minutes to complete crystallization.

CHAPTER 3

Microscale Synthesis

1. MICROSYNTHESIS OF ORGANIC AND MEDICINAL INTERMEDIATES (1–23)

Experiment 1

Aim: To synthesize acetylsalicylic acid (aspirin) on a microscale basis.

General reaction:

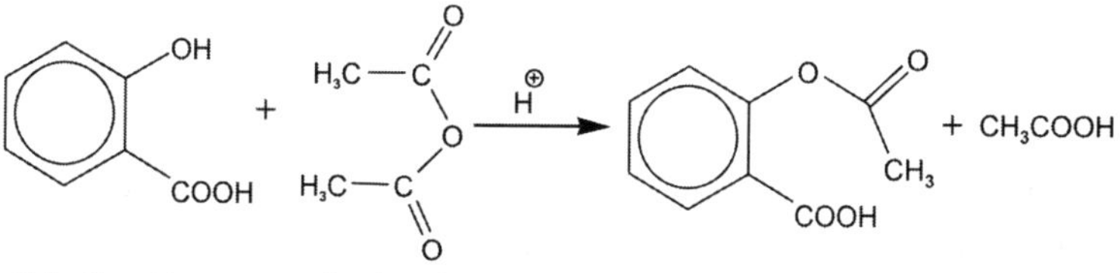

Salicylic acid   Acetic anhydride   Aspirin

Reaction mechanism:

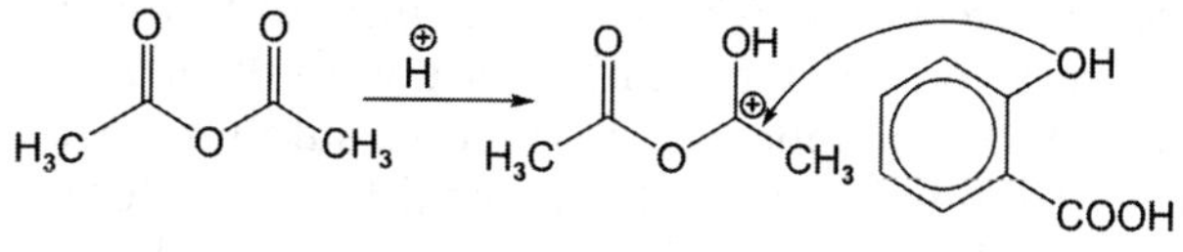

57

Aspirin

Materials:

Chemicals and reagents	Glasswares and equipment
Salicylic acid	Test tube, syringe, glass dropper, 2 beakers, thermometer, boiling chips, Hirsch funnel, filter paper
Acetic anhydride	
Conc. phosphoric acid or conc. sulphuric acid	
Ethanol	
Ice	
Water	

Safety precautions:
- Wear goggles at all times in the lab.
- Acetic anhydride is an irritant and flammable liquid, handle it with care.
- Phosphoric acid and sulphuric acid are very corrosive, handle them with care.

Procedure: Accurately weigh about 140 mg of salicylic acid and place it in a test tube. Add a boiling chip. Add from the side of the test tube, 0.3 ml acetic anhydride with the syringe and one drop of 85% phosphoric acid or conc. sulphuric acid. The acetic anhydride will wash salicylic acid to the bottom of the test tube. Mix the reactants thoroughly and heat the mixture gently by placing it in a beaker of hot (but not boiling) water. The temperature must be around 70–90°C. After 15 minutes of heating, cautiously add 0.2 ml of water to decompose the excess acetic anhydride. When no more evidence of reaction is observed, add 0.3 ml more water; remove the tube from the hot water bath and allow it to cool slowly to room temperature. If crystallization does not occur spontaneously, add a seed crystal or scratch the inside of the tube with a stirring rod. Cool the tube in a beaker of ice water for several minutes until crystallization is complete. Collect the crystals of acetylsalicylic acid by vacuum filtration with a Hirsch funnel and wash the product with only 2–3 ml of ice water and recrystallize from ethanol. Filter and dry the pure crystals on a piece of filter paper and then allow it to dry thoroughly in air before weighing. Determine the yield of the product. Check its purity by measuring the melting point and comparing it with the literature value. Also, record the TLC and IR of the product.

Observation:

Salicylic acid used:	_____ mg
Filter paper:	_____ mg
Filter paper and product:	_____ mg
Dry product:	_____ mg

Calculation:

Mol. formula:	$C_7H_6O_3$	$C_9H_8O_4$
Mol. weight (g/mol):	138	180

138 g : 0.14 g : 180 g?

0.14 × 180/138 = 0.182 g or 182 mg (theoretical yield)

182 mg : y mg : 100%

'y' × 100/182 = _____ % (practical yield)

Where 'y' = practical yield

Result:

1. The m.p/b.p of the product was found to be _____.
2. The R_f value in the used mobile phase was found to be _____.

3. The % yield of the crude and purified product was found to be _____ and _____ respectively.

> **Note:** The calculations are shown in this experiment only. The students should calculate the same for other given experiments using the same methodology.

Experiment 2

Aim: To synthesize 5-nitro salicylic acid on a microscale basis.

General reaction:

Salicylic acid   5-nitro salicylic acid

Reaction mechanism:

Materials:

Chemicals and reagents	Glasswares and equipment
Salicylic acid	Round bottom flask (5 ml), condenser, boiling chip, Hickman head, Guard tube, Test tube (5 ml), Hirsch funnel, filter paper
Conc. sulphuric acid (H_2SO_4)	
Conc. nitric acid (HNO_3)	
Ice	
Water	

Safety precautions:

- Wear goggles, gloves and face mask at all times in the lab.
- Salicylic acid is irritant to skin and eyes, handle it with care.
- The concentrated acids used are corrosive and their vapours are toxic, hence needs to be handled with care.

Procedure: Carefully mix 1 ml of conc. HNO_3 and 1 ml of conc. H_2SO_4 in a 5 ml round bottom flask and add a boiling chip. Attach a Hickman head, condenser and a guard tube to it. On heating with free flame, fumes of nitric acid will be collected in the Hickman head. Then transfer about 0.5 ml of this mixed acid to 200 mg of salicylic acid taken in a test tube, mix well and cool in an ice bath. Allow to stand for about 20 minutes and pour the acid solution over 2–3 ml of ice cold water. Filter the yellowish solid on Hirsch funnel, wash with water (twice with 5 ml) and recrystallize from water. Determine the yield of the product. Check its purity by measuring the melting point and comparing it with the literature value. Also, record the TLC and IR of the product.

Observation:

Salicylic acid used: _____ mg
Filter paper: _____ mg
Filter paper and product: _____ mg
Dry product: _____ mg

Result:

1. The m.p/b.p of the product was found to be _____.

2. The R_f value in the used mobile phase was found to be _____.

3. The % yield of the crude and purified product was found to be _____ and _____ respectively.

Experiment 3

Aim: To synthesize *p*-bromoaniline on microscale basis.

Step 1: Bromination of acetanilide to form p-bromoacetanilide.

General reaction:

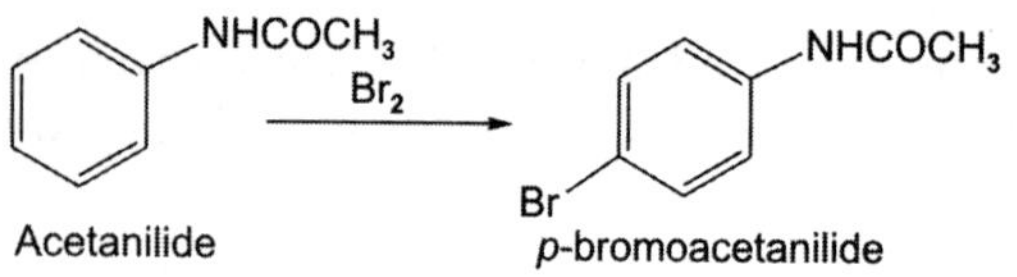

Acetanilide   p-bromoacetanilide

Reaction mechanism:

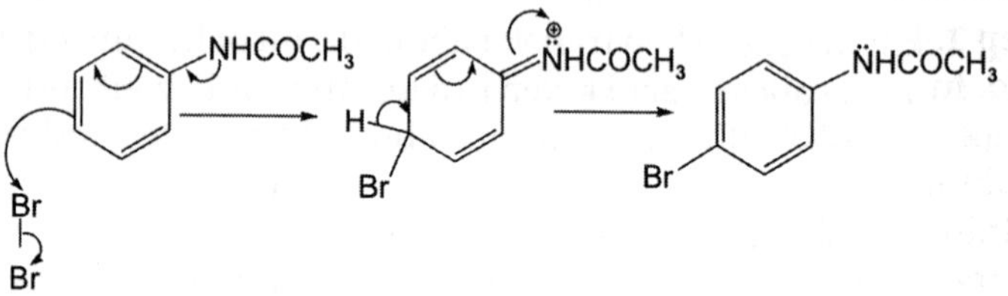

Step 2: Hydrolysis of *p*-bromoacetanilide to *p*-bromoaniline

General reaction:

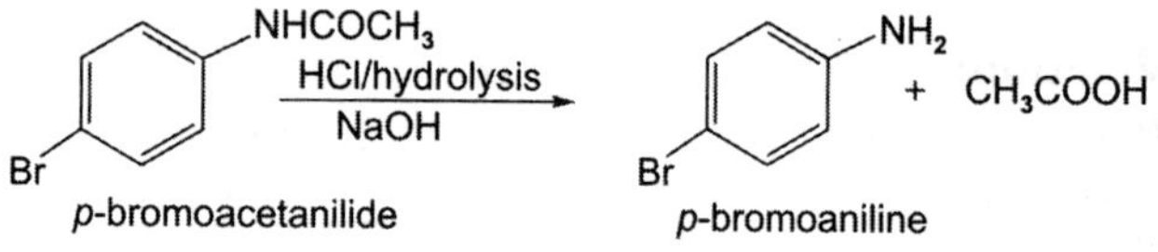

p-bromoacetanilide   p-bromoaniline

Safety precautions: Bromine can cause extreme irritation to the nose, throat and respiratory system at low level vapor exposure. Severe exposures to vapors or contact with bromine solution can cause nose and throat burns, lung inflammation and pulmonary edema. Safety measures mentioned below are to be followed:

- Wear safety goggles at all times in the lab.
- Wear gloves when measuring bromine.
- Addition of bromine should be carried out in fumehood.

Materials:

Chemicals and reagents	Glasswares and equipment
Bromine	Conical flask (10 ml), round bottom flask (5 ml), reflux condenser, Hirsch funnel, drying tube, dropper, fume hood
Acetanilide	
Glacial acetic acid	
Ethanol	
1 N sodium hydroxide (NaOH)	
Hydrochloric acid (HCl)	

Procedure:

Step 1: Dissolve 250 mg of acetanilide in 1 ml of glacial acetic acid. In a 10 ml conical flask, add 0.12 ml of 20 % (v/v) bromine in acetic acid. Allow to stand for 30 minutes with intermittent shaking and swirling. If the initial yellow colour vanishes within first 10 minutes, add another portion of about 0.05 ml of bromine solution. Add 1 ml of water to the mixture, stir well, filter and wash with water (2 × 5 ml) and crystallize from water. Determine the yield of the product. Check its purity by measuring the melting point and comparing it with the literature value. Also, record the TLC and IR of the product.

Step 2: Dissolve 0.2 g of the above product in 1 ml ethanol in a 5 ml round bottom flask. Add 0.25 ml conc. HCl and reflux for 45 minutes. Evaporate ethanol and add 1.5 ml water and make the solution alkaline with dropwise addition of 1 N NaOH with cooling in ice water. Filter and wash with water (twice with 5 ml) and crystallize from water. Determine the yield of the product. Check its purity by measuring the melting point and comparing it with the literature value. Also, record the TLC and IR of the product.

Step 1:
Observation:

Acetanilide:	_____ mg
Filter paper:	_____ mg
Filter paper and product:	_____ mg
Dry product:	_____ mg

Step 2:
Observation:

p-bromo acetanilide:	_____ mg
Filter paper:	_____ mg
Filter paper and product:	_____ mg
Dry product:	_____ mg

Result:

1. The m.p/b.p of the product was found to be _____.
2. The R_f value in the used mobile phase was found to be

   _____.

3. The % yield of the crude and purified product was found to be _____ and _____ respectively.

Experiment 4

Aim: To synthesize benzil on microscale basis.

General reaction:

Benzoin   Benzil

Reaction mechanism:

Safety precautions:
- Wear goggles and gloves at all times in the lab.
- Benzoin is irritant to eyes and skin, hence needs to be handled with care.

Materials:

Chemicals and reagents	Glasswares and equipment
Benzoin	Round bottom flask (10 ml), water bath, Hirsch funnel, beaker (10 ml), filter paper
Conc. nitric acid	
Ice cold water	
Alcohol	

Procedure: Place 300 mg of benzoin and 1.5 ml of conc. nitric acid in a 10 ml round bottom flask. Then heat on a boiling water bath, with occasional shaking for about 1.5 hours. When the evolution of brown gas fumes has ceased, pour the reaction mixture in 5–6 ml cold water in a beaker. Stir till all the product crystallizes as yellow solid. Filter on Hirsch funnel, wash thoroughly with water (2 × 5 ml) to remove the traces of acid and recrystallize from alcohol. Determine the yield of the product. Check its purity by measuring the melting point and comparing it with the literature value. Also, record the TLC and IR of the product.

Observation:

Benzoin: _____ mg

Filter paper: _____ mg

Filter paper and product: _____ mg

Dry product: _____ mg

Result:
1. The m.p/b.p of the product was found to be _____.
2. The R_f value in the used mobile phase was found to be _____.
3. The % yield of the crude and purified product was found to be _____ and _____ respectively.

Experiment 5

Aim: To synthesize benzilic acid on microscale basis.

General reaction:

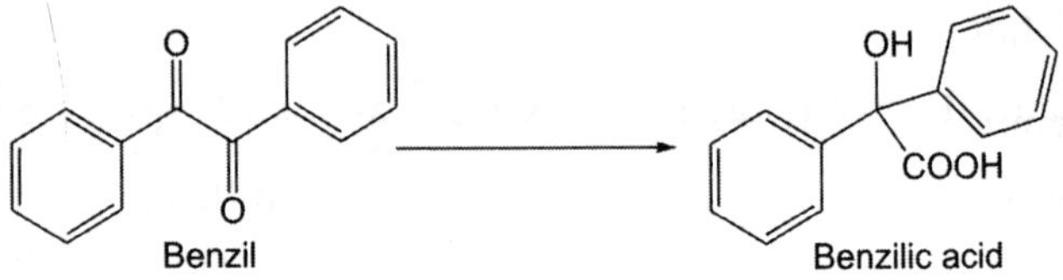

Benzil → Benzilic acid

Reaction mechanism:

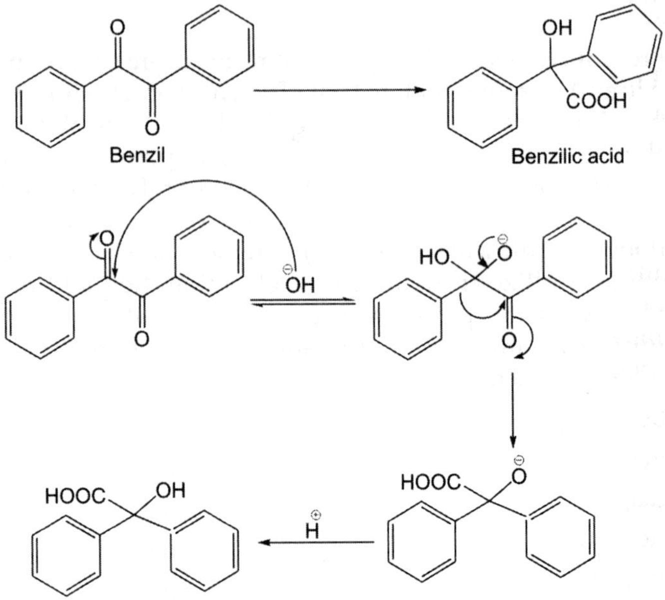

Benzil → Benzilic acid

Safety precautions:
- Wear goggles and gloves at all times in the lab.
- Benzil is an irritant although not much toxic.

- Strong alkali like NaOH and strong acids like HCl are toxic and corrosive, hence needed to be handled with care.

Materials:

Chemicals and reagents	Glasswares and equipment
Benzil	Round bottom flask (10 ml), reflux condenser, Hirsch funnel, beaker (10 ml), dropper, filter paper
Potassium hydroxide	
Conc. Hydrochloric acid (HCl)	
Congo red paper	

Procedure: Reflux a mixture of 100 mg of benzil, 350 mg of potassium hydroxide in 4 ml of water and 4 ml ethanol for about 15 minutes. Cool thoroughly till the potassium benzilate salt precipitates. Dissolve the salt in about 2 ml of water and neutralize by dropwise addition of conc. HCl till acidic to Congo red paper. Filter on Hirsch funnel, wash with water (2 × 5 ml) and recrystallize from water. Determine the yield of the product. Check its purity by measuring the melting point and comparing it with the literature value. Also, record the TLC and IR of the product.

Observation:

Benzil: _____ mg

Filter paper: _____ mg

Filter paper and product: _____ mg

Dry product: _____ mg

Result:

1. The m.p/b.p of the product was found to be _____.

2. The R_f value in the used mobile phase was found to be _____.

3. The % yield of the crude and purified product was found to be _____ and _____ respectively.

Experiment 6

Aim: To synthesize 2,3-diphenyl quinoxaline on a microscale basis.

Benzil

Benzil quinoxaline

Reaction:

Chemicals and reagents	Glasswares and equipment
Benzil	Conical flask (10 ml), Hirsch funnel, beaker (10 ml)
o-phenylenediamine	
Alcohol	

Materials:

Safety precautions:

- Wear goggles and gloves at all times in the lab.
- Benzil is an irritant although not much toxic but o-phenylenediamine is an extremely toxic and carcinogenic compound. Hence it should be handled with care.

Procedure: Add 100 mg of benzil and 100 mg o-phenylenediamine to 5 ml of alcohol in a conical vial and warm it slightly. On cooling, quinoxaline product precipitates out. Filter on Hirsch funnel, wash with water (2 × 5 ml) and recrystallize from alcohol. Record the yield of the product. Check its purity by measuring the melting point and compare it with the literature value.

Observation:

Benzil used:	_____	mg
Filter paper:	_____	mg
Filter paper and product:	_____	mg
Dry product:	_____	mg

Result:

1. The m.p/b.p of the product was found to be _____.

2. The R_f value in the used mobile phase was found to be _____.

3. The % yield of the crude and purified product was found to be _____ and _____ respectively.

Experiment 7

Aim: To synthesize 9,10-dihydroanthracene-9,10-succinic anhydride on microscale basis.

General reaction:

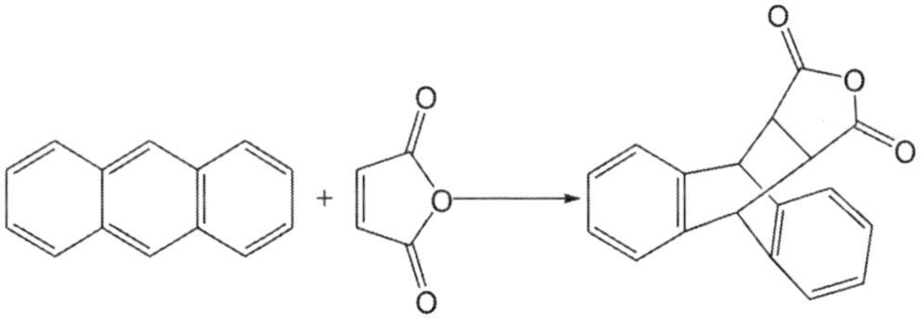

Anthracene   Maleic anhydride   9,10-dihydroanthracene-9,10-succinic acid anhydride

Reaction mechanism:

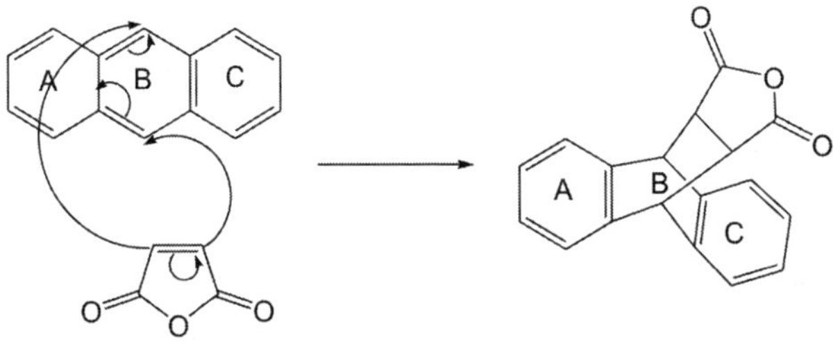

Safety precautions:

• Wear goggles and face mask at all times in the lab.

• Anthracene and maleic anhydride are irritant and toxic to eyes and skin, while the latte causes burns too. Hence should be handled with care.

• Solvents like toluene and petroleum ether are irritant and toxic upon inhalation.

Materials:

Chemicals and reagents	Glasswares and equipment
Anthracene	Round bottom flask (5 ml), reflux condenser, Hirsch funnel, beaker (10 ml), guard tube
Maleic anhydride	
Toluene (dry)	
Calcium carbonate	
Petroleum ether	
Alcohol	

Procedure: Reflux a solution of 80 mg of anthracene and 40 mg of maleic anhydride in less than 1 ml of dry toluene in a 5 ml round bottom flask equipped with condenser and a guard tube (with calcium carbonate or calcium chloride) for about 30 minutes. Cool and hold the flask in ice cold water when solid separates. Filter on Hirsch funnel, wash with petroleum ether (2 × 5 ml) and recrystallize from alcohol. Determine the yield of the product. Check its purity by measuring the melting point and comparing it with the literature value. Also, record the TLC and IR of the product.

Observation:

Anthracene: _____ mg

Filter paper: _____ mg

Filter paper and product: _____ mg

Dry product: _____ mg

Result:

1. The m.p/b.p of the product was found to be _____.

2. The R_f value in the used mobile phase was found to be _____.

3. The % yield of the crude and purified product was found to be _____ and _____ respectively.

Experiment 8

Aim: To synthesize quinone on microscale basis.

General reaction:

Reaction mechanism:

Safety precautions:
- Wear goggles at all times in the lab.
- Hydroquinone and potassium bromated are irritant and toxic, while the latter is carcinogenic too. Hence should be handled with care.

Materials:

Chemicals and reagents	Glasswares and equipments
Hydroquinone	Round bottom flask (10 ml), reflux condenser, Hirsch funnel, beaker (10 ml), water bath
Dil. sulphuric acid (H_2SO_4)	
Potassium bromate	

Procedure: Dissolve 250 mg of hydroquinone in 2.5 ml of water at 50°C in a 10 ml round bottom flask attached with a condenser. Cool the solution to room temperature when hydroquinone is completely dissolved. Then add 1 ml of dil. H_2SO_4 and 140 mg of potassium bromate in three portions. Heat around 60°C on water bath for 10 minutes. Cool in ice.

Yellow crystals of quinine will begin to precipitate. Filter on Hirsch funnel, wash with water (2 × 5 ml) and recrystallize from water.

Observation:

Hydroquinone:	_____ mg
Filter paper:	_____ mg
Filter paper and product:	_____ mg
Dry product:	_____ mg

Result:

1. The m.p/b.p of the product was found to be _____.
2. The R_f value in the used mobile phase was found to be

   _____.

3. The % yield of the crude and purified product was found to be _____ and _____ respectively.

Experiment 9

Aim: To synthesize benzalacetophenone on microscale basis.

General reaction:

| Benzaldehyde | Acetophenone | Benzalacetophenone |

Reaction mechanism:

Safety precautions:
- Wear goggles and face masks at all times in the lab.
- Acetophenone and benzaldehyde are irritant, flammable and toxic to inhale, hence handle it with care.

Materials:

Chemicals and reagents	Glasswares and equipment
Acetophenone	Conical flask (10 ml), Hirsch funnel, beaker (10 ml)
Benzaldehyde	
Sodium hydroxide (NaOH)	
Ethanol	

Procedure: Mix 250 mg of acetophenone and 110 mg of NaOH in 2 ml water and 1.5 ml ethanol to make a homogeneous solution. Then add 0.25 ml of benzaldehyde and stir the mixture at room temperature with a glass rod till a thick paste is formed. Leave it overnight and then filter on Hirsch funnel. Wash with cold water (2 × 5 ml) and recrystallize from ethanol.

Observation:

Acetophenone: _____ mg

Filter paper: _____ mg

Filter paper and product: _____ mg

Dry product: _____ mg

Result:

1. The m.p/b.p of the product was found to be _____.

2. The R_f value in the used mobile phase was found to be _____.

3. The % yield of the crude and purified product was found to be _____ and _____ respectively.

Experiment 10

Aim: To synthesize benzhydrol on microscale basis.

Reaction:

Benzophenone   Zn/NaOH   Benzhydrol

Safety precautions:
- Wear goggles and face masks at all times in the lab.
- Benzophenone and sodium hydroxide are irritant to eyes, skin and mucous membrane, toxic to ingest, hence handle it with care.
- Conc. HCl is extremely toxic and corrosive, hence handle it with care.

Materials:

Chemicals and reagents	Glasswares and equipment
Benzophenone	Conical flask (10 ml), Hirsch funnel, beaker (10 ml)
Sodium hydroxide	
Zinc dust	
Ethanol	
Conc. HCl	

Procedure: Prepare a solution of 125 mg of pure benzophenone in 1.5 ml of ethanol in a conical flask. To it, add 125 mg sodium hydroxide and 125 mg of zinc dust. Shake the contents of the flask and warm at around 70°C for 90 minutes. Allow the reaction mixture to cool when solid separates. Filter on Hirsch funnel, wash the residue with hot ethanol (2 × 5 ml).

Pour the filtrate in 5 ml ice cold water and acidify by adding conc. HCl with a dropper. The product separates as a viscous oil and solidifies after standing overnight. Filter on Hirsch funnel and recrystallize from ethanol. Record the yield of the product. Check its purity by measuring the melting point and compare it with the literature value.

Observation:

Benzophenone:	_____ mg
Filter paper:	_____ mg
Filter paper and product:	_____ mg
Dry product:	_____ mg

Result:

1. The m.p/b.p of the product was found to be _____.
2. The R_f value in the used mobile phase was found to be _____.
3. The % yield of the crude and purified product was found to be _____ and _____ respectively.

Experiment 11

Aim: To synthesize phenothiazine on microscale basis.

Reaction:

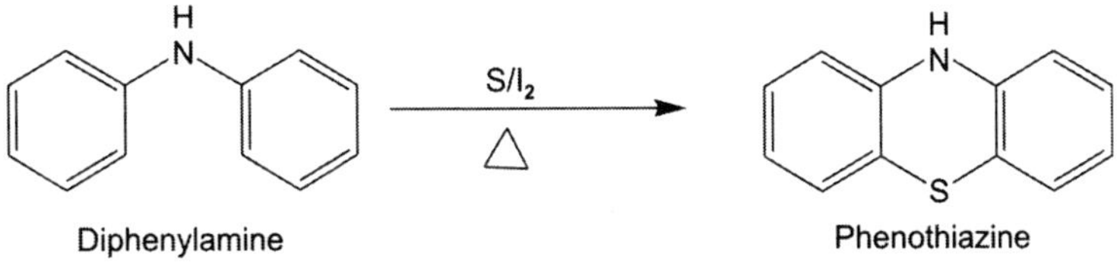

Diphenylamine S/I_2, $\triangle$ Phenothiazine

Safety precautions:
• Wear goggles and face masks at all times in the lab.

- Diphenylamine, sulphur and iodine irritant to eyes, skin and mucous membrane, toxic to ingest, hence handle it with care.

Materials:

Chemicals and reagents	Glasswares and equipment
Diphenylamine	Conical flask (10 ml), Hirsch funnel, beaker (10 ml)
Sulphur	
Iodine	

Procedure: Take 300 mg of diphenyl amine, 100 mg sulphur powder and 50 mg iodine. Heat the mixture on sand bath for about 10 minutes. Cool to room temperature, add 2.5–4 ml of ethanol and heat again on sand bath till the solution is clear. Filter on Hirsch funnel and recrystallize from ethanol. Record the yield of the product. Check its purity by measuring the melting point and compare it with the literature value.

Observation:

Diphenylamine: _____ mg

Filter paper: _____ mg

Filter paper and product: _____ mg

Dry product: _____ mg

Result:

1. The m.p/b.p of the product was found to be _____.

2. The R_f value in the used mobile phase was found to be _____.

3. The % yield of the crude and purified product was found to be _____ and _____ respectively.

Experiment 12

Aim: To synthesize 7-hydroxy-4-methyl coumarin on microscale basis.

Reaction:

7-hydroxy-4-methyl coumarin

Safety precautions:

- Wear goggles and face masks at all times in the lab.
- Resorcinol, urea and sodium hydroxide are irritant to eyes, skin and mucous membrane, toxic to ingest, hence handle it with care.
- Ethyl acetoacetate and polyphosphoric acid are toxic to inhale and latter is extremely corrosive, hence handle it with care.

Materials:

Chemicals and reagents	Glasswares and equipment
Resorcinol	Conical flask (10 ml), Hirsch funnel, beaker (10 ml)
Ethyl acetoacetate	
Polyphosphoric acid	
Ethanol	

Procedure: Prepare a solution of 140 mg of resorcinol and 5 drops of ethyl acetoacetate in a conical flask. Add 1 ml of cold conc. sulphuric acid to it and heat the reaction mixture on water bath for 20 minutes. Add about 5 ml of ice-cold water to it when pale yellow solid precipitates out. Filter on Hirsch funnel, wash with 5 ml of water and recrystallize from dilute methanol. Record the yield of the product. Check its purity by measuring the melting point and compare it with the literature value.

Observation:

Resorcinol:	_____ mg
Filter paper:	_____ mg
Filter paper and product:	_____ mg
Dry product:	_____ mg

Result:

1. The m.p/b.p of the product was found to be _____.
2. The R_f value in the used mobile phase was found to be
   _____.
3. The % yield of the crude and purified product was found to be _____ and _____ respectively.

Experiment 13

Aim: To synthesize benzimidazole microscale basis.

o-phenylenediamine

Cyclization

Benzimidazole

Reaction:

Safety precautions:

- Wear goggles and face masks at all times in the lab.
- O-phenylene diamine is extremely toxic and carcinogenic compound, hence handle it with care.
- Formic acid and sodium hydroxide are irritant to skin, mucous membrane and toxic to inhale, hence handle it with care.

Materials:

Chemicals and reagents	Glasswares and equipment
o-lhenylene diamine	Conical flask (10 ml), Hirsch funnel, beaker (10 ml)
Formic acid	
Sodium hydroxide	
Ethanol	

Procedure: Heat a mixture of 270 mg of o-phenylenediamine and 175 mg of 90% formic acid in a 5 ml round bottom flask on a water bath for 2 hours. Cool the mixture and add 15 % NaOH solution with constant stirring (magnetic or manual) till the mixture is just alkaline to litmus paper when solid separates. Filter on Hirsch funnel, add the filtered crude product and 10 mg of charcoal in 10 ml of boiling water. Again filter on Hirsch funnel, wash with 5 ml of cold water and recrystallize from dilute ethanol. Determine the yield of the product. Check its purity by measuring the melting point and comparing it with the literature value. Also, record the TLC and IR of the product.

Observation:

o-phenylenediamine: _____ mg

Filter paper: _____ mg

Filter paper and product: _____ mg

Dry product: _____ mg

Result:

1. The m.p/b.p of the product was found to be _____.

2. The R_f value in the used mobile phase was found to be _____.

3. The % yield of the crude and purified product was found to be _____ and _____ respectively.

Experiment 14

Aim: To synthesize phenytoin on microscale basis.

Reaction:

Safety precautions:

- Wear goggles and face masks at all times in the lab.
- Benzil, urea and sodium hydroxide are irritant to eyes, skin and mucous membrane, toxic to ingest, hence handle it with care.

Materials:

Chemicals and reagents	Glasswares and equipment
Benzil	Conical flask (10 ml), Hirsch funnel, beaker (10 ml)
Urea	
Ethanol	
Sodium hydroxide	
Conc. HCl	

Procedure: Reflux a mixture of 500 mg benzil and 250 mg urea in 7.5 ml of ethanol and 1.5 ml of 30% aqueous NaOH solution in a conical flask for around 2 hours. Cool the flask and add 2 ml of ice cold water to it when solid separates after a few minutes. Filter on Hirsch funnel to remove insoluble impurity. Add conc. HCl dropwise through a dropper to the filtrate till just acidic when the product precipitates out. Filter on Hirsch funnel, wash with 5 ml cold water and recrystallize from dilute ethanol. Determine the yield of the product. Check its purity

by measuring the melting point and comparing it with the
literature value. Also, record the TLC and IR of the product.

Observation:

Benzil:	_____ mg
Filter paper:	_____ mg
Filter paper and product:	_____ mg
Dry product:	_____ mg

Result:

1. The m.p/b.p of the product was found to be _____.
2. The R_f value in the used mobile phase was found to be
   _____.
3. The % yield of the crude and purified product was found
   to be _____ and _____ respectively.

Experiment 15

Aim: To synthesize paracetamol on microscale basis.

Reaction:

| p-amino phenol | Acetic anhydride | Paracetamol |

Safety precautions:

- Wear goggles and face masks at all times in the lab.
- Acetic anhydride and conc. sulphuric acid are irritant,
  corrosive and toxic to inhale, hence handle it with care.
- *p*-amino phenol when accidently ingested can cause
  nephrotoxicity and hepatotoxicity.

Materials:

Chemicals and reagents	Glasswares and equipment
p-amino phenol	Conical flask (10 ml), Hirsch funnel, beaker (10 ml)
Acetic anhydride	
conc. sulphuric acid	
Ethanol	
Charcoal	

Procedure: Take 600 mg of p-amino phenol in a conical flask. Add 0.65 ml of acetic anhydride and 1 drop of conc. sulphuric acid to it. The reaction mixture is warmed on water bath at around 60°C with constant stirring for 30 minutes. Allow the reaction mixture to cool to room temperature. Add about 3 ml of ice-cold water to it when solid precipitates out. Filter on Hirsch funnel, wash with 5 ml of water. Recrystallization is performed by dissolving the crude product in 70% ethanol, adding 10 mg of charcoal and warming it to 70°C. The mixture is again filtered on Hirsch funnel. The filtrate is concentrated over a water bath when pure crystals of product separate out. Record the yield of the product. Check its purity by measuring the melting point and compare it with the literature value.

Observation:

p-amino phenol: _____ mg

Filter paper: _____ mg

Filter paper and product: _____ mg

Dry product: _____ mg

Result:

1. The m.p/b.p of the product was found to be _____.

2. The R_f value in the used mobile phase was found to be _____.

3. The % yield of the crude and purified product was found to be _____ and _____ respectively.

Experiment 16

Aim: To synthesize acetanilide on microscale basis.

Reaction:

| Aniline | Acetic anhydride | Acetanilide |

Safety precautions:
- Wear goggles and face masks at all times in the lab.
- Aniline and sodium acetate are skin irritant, hence handle it with care.
- Conc. hydrochloric acid and acetic anhydride are irritant, corrosive and toxic to inhale, hence handle it with care.

Materials:

Chemicals and reagents	Glasswares and equipment
Aniline	Conical flask (10 ml), Hirsch funnel, beaker (10 ml)
Conc. hydrochloric acid	
Acetic anhydride	
Sodium acetate	
Ethanol	

Procedure: Prepare a solution of 1 ml of aniline in 0.6 ml of conc. HCl and 2 ml of water in a 10 ml round bottom flask by stirring. Then add 2 ml of acetic anhydride to this reaction mixture and stir to dissolve. Then pour this mixture in a solution of 1.5 g of sodium acetate in 5 ml of water. Stir this mixture vigorously and keep in ice bath. The crude product crystallizes as white solid. Filter on Hirsch funnel, wash thoroughly with water (2×5 ml) and recrystallize from dilute ethanol. The product is obtained as white glistening crystals. Determine the yield of the product. Check its purity by measuring the melting point and comparing it with the literature value. Also, record the TLC and IR of the product.

Observation:

Aniline:	_____ mg
Filter paper:	_____ mg
Filter paper and product:	_____ mg
Dry product:	_____ mg

Result:

1. The m.p/b.p of the product was found to be _____.
2. The R_f value in the used mobile phase was found to be _____.
3. The % yield of the crude and purified product was found to be _____ and _____ respectively.

Experiment 17

Aim: To synthesize benzanilide on microscale basis.

Reaction:

| Aniline | Benzoyl chloride | Benzanilide |

Safety precautions:

- Wear goggles and face masks at all times in the lab.
- Aniline and sodium hydroxide are skin irritant, hence handle it with care.

- Benzoyl chloride is irritant to eyes, skin and toxic to inhale, hence handle it with care.

Materials:

Chemicals and reagents	Glasswares and equipment
Aniline	Conical flask (10 ml), Hirsch funnel, beaker (10 ml)
Sodium hydroxide	
Benzoyl chloride	
Ethanol	

Procedure: Prepare a solution of 260 mg of aniline in 2.5 ml of 10 % aqueous NaOH solution in a conical flask. Then add 5–6 drops of benzoyl chloride and stopper the flask. Shake vigorously for about 10 minutes. The reaction mixture becomes hot as it evolves heat. The completion of reaction is indicated by disappearance of odour of benzoyl chloride when white coloured separates out. Then add 2 ml of water to the reaction mass. Filter on Hirsch funnel, wash with 5 ml of water and recrystallize from dilute ethanol. Record the yield of the product. Check its purity by measuring the melting point and compare it with the literature value.

Observation:

Aniline:	_____mg
Filter paper:	_____mg
Filter paper and product:	_____mg
Dry product:	_____mg

Result:

1. The m.p/b.p of the product was found to be _____.
2. The R_f value in the used mobile phase was found to be _____.
3. The % yield of the crude and purified product was found to be _____ and _____ respectively.

Experiment 18

Aim: To synthesize 1,1'-bisnaphthol on microscale basis.

General reaction:

Beta naphthol

1,1'-bis-2,2'-naphthol

Safety precautions:
- Wear goggles and face masks at all times in the lab.
- b-naphthol and ferric chloride are irritant to skin and mucous membrane, toxic to ingest, hence handle it with care.

Materials:

Chemicals and reagents	Glasswares and equipment
β-naphthol	Conical flask (10 ml), Hirsch funnel, beaker (10 ml)
Ferric chloride	
Water	
Ethanol	

Procedure: Place 200 mg of β-naphthol in a conical flask and add 5 ml of water to it. Attach a condenser and reflux until the reaction mixture starts boiling and as suspension of β-naphthol is formed. Separately prepare a solution of 400 mg of ferric chloride in 2 ml of water. Add this solution to the reaction mixture and continue boiling further for about 10 minutes. The oily droplets disappear and the product separates out. Filter on Hirsch funnel, wash with water (2 × 5 ml) and recrystallize from ethanol. Determine the yield of the product. Check its purity by measuring the melting point and comparing it with the literature value. Also, record the TLC and IR of the product.

Observation:

β-naphthol: _____ mg
Filter paper: _____ mg
Filter paper and product: _____ mg
Dry product: _____ mg

Result:

1. The m.p/b.p of the product was found to be _____.
2. The R_f value in the used mobile phase was found to be

   _____.

3. The % yield of the crude and purified product was found to be _____ and _____ respectively.

Experiment 19

Aim: To synthesize benzamide on microscale basis.

Reaction:

Benzoyl chloride   Penzamide

Safety precautions:

• Wear goggles and face masks at all times in the lab.
• Benzoyl chloride and ammonia are irritant to eyes, skin and toxic to inhale, hence handle it with care.

Materials:

Chemicals and reagents	Glasswares and equipment
conc. ammonia solution	Conical flask (10 ml), Hirsch funnel, beaker (10 ml)
Benzoyl chloride	

Procedure: Place 1 ml of conc. ammonia solution in a conical vial and add 0.2 ml of benzoyl chloride to it by means of a dropper shaking the vial frequently. Drop by drop addition should be made for a period of 2–3 minutes when the product separates out. Filter on Hirsch funnel, wash with 5 ml of cold water and recrystallize from water. Determine the yield of the product. Check its purity by measuring the melting point and comparing it with the literature value. Also, record the TLC and IR of the product.

Observation:

Benzoyl chloride: _____ mg
Filter paper: _____ mg
Filter paper and product: _____ mg
Dry product: _____ mg

Result:

1. The m.p/b.p of the product was found to be _____.
2. The R_f value in the used mobile phase was found to be

_____.

3. The % yield of the crude and purified product was found to be _____ and _____ respectively.

Experiment 20

Aim: To synthesize 5,5-diphenyl-2-thioimidazolin-4-one on microscale basis.

Reaction:

Benzil   Thiourea   5,5-diphenyl-2-
                                            thioimidazolin-4-one

Safety precautions:

- Wear goggles and face masks at all times in the lab.
- Benzil, thiourea and sodium hydroxide are irritants although not much toxic.
- Conc. HCl is irritant, corrosive and toxic to inhale, hence handle with care.

Materials:

Chemicals and reagents	Glasswares and equipment
Benzil	Conical flask (10 ml), Hirsch funnel, beaker (10 ml)
Thiourea	
Sodium hydroxide	
Ethanol	
conc. HCl	
Water	

Procedure: Place 350 mg of benzil, 200 mg of thiourea, 1 ml of aqueous NaOH and 5 ml of ethanol in a 10 ml round bottom flask. Attach it to a reflux condenser and boil for 2 hours. Cool the reaction mixture to room temperature and pour it into 10 ml of water. Mix thoroughly and allow to stand or 15 minutes and filter under suction. Collect the filtrate, cool it in ice bath and acidify with conc. HCl. Filter on Hirsch funnel, wash thoroughly with 5 ml of water and recrystallize from ethanol. Determine the yield of the product. Check its purity by measuring the melting point and comparing it with the literature value. Also, record the TLC and IR of the product.

Observation:

Benzil:	_____	mg
Filter paper:	_____	mg
Filter paper and product:	_____	mg
Dry product:	_____	mg

Result:

1. The m.p/b.p of the product was found to be _____.

2. The R_f value in the used mobile phase was found to be

   _____.

3. The % yield of the crude and purified product was found
   to be _____ and _____ respectively.

Experiment 21

Aim: To synthesize benzotriazole on microscale basis.

Reaction:

o-phenylene diamine   Benzotriazole

Safety precautions:

- Wear goggles and face masks at all times in the lab.

- o-phenylene diamine is extremely toxic and carcinogenic
  compound and sodium nitrite is toxic when exposed to
  skin, hence handle it with care.

- Glacial acetic acid and benzene are irritant to skin,
  mucous membrane and toxic to inhale, hence handle it
  with care.

Materials:

Chemicals and reagents	Glasswares and equipment
o-phenylene diamine	Conical flask (10 ml), Hirsch funnel, beaker (10 ml)
Glacial acetic acid	
Sodium nitrite	
Water	
Benzene	

Procedure: Place 110 mg of *o*-phenylene diamine, 2 drops of glacial acetic acid and 7 drops of water in a conical flask and warm the mixture if required. Prepare a solution of 750 mg of sodium nitrite in 0.15 ml of water separately in a beaker and cool it in ice bath to reach the temperature around 0–5°C. Add this cold sodium nitrite solution to the reaction mixture. Then warm the reaction mixture with stirring such that a temperature of 85°C is attained in 2–3 minutes and then begin to cool. The white colour of the mixture changes from deep blue to pale brown. Stirring is continued for further 15 minutes by which time the temperature drops down to 35–40°C. Then the mixture is thoroughly in ice bath for about 30 minutes. Filter the separated pale brown solid on Hirsch funnel, wash thoroughly with 5 ml of water and recrystallize from benzene. Determine the yield of the product. Check its purity by measuring the melting point and comparing it with the literature value. Also, record the TLC and IR of the product.

Observation:

o-phenylene diamine:	_____ mg
Filter paper:	_____ mg
Filter paper and product:	_____ mg
Dry product:	_____ mg

Result:

1. The m.p/b.p of the product was found to be _____.
2. The R_f value in the used mobile phase was found to be _____.
3. The % yield of the crude and purified product was found to be _____ and _____ respectively.

Experiment 22

Aim: To synthesize o-iodo benzoic acid on microscale basis.

Reaction:

Safety precautions:

Anthranilic acid → (NaNO₂/H₂SO₄, ice bath) → Diazo salt → (KI, Δ) → o-iodo benzoic acid

- Wear goggles and face masks at all times in the lab.
- Anthranilic acid is extremely irritant to skin, and mucous membrane, while sodium nitrite and potassium iodide are less irritant, but handle it with care.

Materials:
Procedure: Dissolve 350 mg of anthranilic acid in 2 ml of

Chemicals and reagents	Glasswares and equipment
Anthranilic acid	Conical flask (10 ml), Hirsch funnel, beaker (10 ml)
Conc. sulphuric acid	
Sodium nitrite	
Potassium iodide	

conc. sulphuric acid. Separately prepare a solution of 200 mg of sodium nitrite in 2 ml of water in a beaker and place it in ice. Then diazotize the acidic mixture of anthranilic acid, by adding cold solution of sodium nitrite to it. Keep the reaction mixture in ice bath for 2–3 minutes. Meanwhile, prepare a solution of 600 mg of potassium iodide in 10 ml of water. Add this solution to the reaction mixture and heat on water bath for 15 minutes and cool again. Dark coloured precipitate of crude product separates out. Filter on Hirsch funnel, wash with cold water (2 × 5 ml) and recrystallize from water. Determine the yield of the product. Check its purity by measuring the melting point and comparing it with the literature value. Also, record the TLC and IR of the product.

Observation:

Anthranilic acid: _____ mg

Filter paper: _____ mg

Filter paper and product: _____ mg

Dry product: _____ mg

Result:

1. The m.p/b.p of the product was found to be _____.
2. The R_f value in the used mobile phase was found to be _____.
3. The % yield of the crude and purified product was found to be _____ and _____ respectively.

Experiment 23

Aim: To synthesize phthalimide on microscale basis.

Reaction:

| Phthalic anhydride | Urea | Phthalimide |

Safety precautions:
- Wear goggles and face masks at all times in the lab.
- Urea and phthalic anhydride are irritant to eyes, skin and mucous membrane, toxic to ingest, hence handle it with care.

Materials:

Chemicals and reagents	Glasswares and equipment
Phthalic anhydride	Conical flask (10 ml), Hirsch funnel, beaker (10 ml)
Urea	
Water	

Procedure: Place 500 mg of phthalic anhydride and 100 mg of urea in a conical flask. Heat the reaction mixture on sand bath at 180°C till 10 minutes or when the volume of reaction mixture increases by approximate 3 times its original volume or when effervescence occur. Then add 5 ml of ice cold water. Filter on

Hirsch funnel, wash with cold water (2 × 5 ml) and recrystallize from ethanol. Determine the yield of the product. Check its purity by measuring the melting point and comparing it with the literature value. Also, record the TLC and IR of the product.

Observation:

Phthalic anhydride: _____ mg

Filter paper: _____ mg

Filter paper and product: _____ mg

Dry product: _____ mg

Result:
1. The m.p/b.p of the product was found to be _____.
2. The R_f value in the used mobile phase was found to be _____.
3. The % yield of the crude and purified product was found to be _____ and _____ respectively.

2. BENEFITS OF MICROSCALE SYNTHESIS

1. In microscale experiments, as the chemicals used are in very small quantity, there is tremendous reduction in fumes and the risks of accidents, chemical spills, acid burns, exposure to toxic chemicals and other related hazards thereby improving laboratory safety.

2. Due to usage of small quantities of chemicals, it lowers the cost for chemical substances and equipment and reduces laboratory cost.

3. It reduces waste at the source and lowers glass breakage cost.

4. It also reduces dependence on intensive ventilation systems causing a significant reduction in electricity consumption.

5. Conducting microscale experiments also saves storage space as it requires smaller storage area.

6. The experiments are quick to perform offering shorter reaction times.

7. Due to less time required for microscale experiment, students can perform more experiments during the saved time to help in better conceptual understanding.

8. Disposal is very easy nearly because all the chemicals can be wiped off with a paper towel which can be placed in a bowl or the bin.

9. They can often take place in a room which is not a set up as a laboratory and even a bucket of water is sufficient.

10. The results can be filmed or photographed on mobile phones (if they are allowed) and can be projected onto screens with web cams, video microscopes or camcorders

11. Student find the working process easy and interesting so that they can concentrate more on the observations.

12. It can be carried out by students working on their own and the experiments can often be carried out sitting down which results in greater control of the class.

CHAPTER 4

Applications

1. MICROSCALE AND MICROWAVE CHEMISTRY

Many organic reactions require heat in order to proceed. In the lab, this is traditionally done using a Bunsen burner, hot plate, steam, oil or sand bath. For those reactions that do require heat, the problem is that these heating sources are inefficient and reactions can often take a long-time to reach completion. By using microwave heating, reaction times can be dramatically reduced and product yields can be higher. Shortening the time of known reactions is not the only advantage that microwave heating is possessing. It is impacting modern organic chemistry by opening up avenues to compounds that were previously not accessible. It is also a cleaner way to do preparative chemistry. Almost any reaction that needs heat can be performed in a microwave. If microwave organic experiments are conducted on a microscale basis, it would naturally make the experiment safer and more cost-effective.

2. MICROSCALE AND GREEN CHEMISTRY

We know that green chemistry emphasizes the concepts of atom economy, source reduction, pathway modification, solvent substitution, and pollution prevention as a means of improving the environmental impact of industrial chemistry. Microscale chemistry can serve as a tool for incorporating green chemistry ideas across the curriculum in the educational institutions. This is because it is performed by using extremely less mounts of chemicals and employing safe and easy techniques through the use of miniature laboratory glassware.

CHAPTER 5

Future Opportunities

With the attributes and benefits of microscale organic synthesis discussed previously, it is not surprising that it has spread like wildfire mainly in developing countries. It has also developed profound roots throughout the world which will make the tree grow quite high for the years to come. Both developed and underdeveloped countries will continue benefiting from this approach.

There are further many advantages of combining microscale chemistry with green chemistry and microwave-assisted organic synthesis because all of these have a common objective of reducing chemical risks. Together, all these techniques represent an effective approach to education and training in chemistry at all levels. Also, advances in current experimental organic chemistry can be achieved and skills can be developed by hands on experience by using special equipment, methods and studying reactions at a deeper level. This technique shall also become a landmark for scale-up of intermediates and reagents in the research and development.

Further Reading

1. Dana W. Mayo, Ronald M. Pike & David C. Forbes. Microscale organic laboratory: With multistep and multiscale syntheses, John Wiley & Sons, 2000. (ISBN-10: 0471215023)
2. Dana Mayo, Ronald Pike, Peter Trumper. Microscale techniques for organic laboratory, John Wiley & Sons, 2001. (ISBN-10: 0471621927)
3. John C. Gilbert, SF Martin. Experimental organic chemistry: A Miniscale and microscale approach, Brooks Cole Publishers, 2015, (ISBN-10: 1439049149)

Index